RAND

Estimating Eye Care Provider Supply and Workforce Requirements

Paul P. Lee, Catherine A. Jackson,
Daniel A. Relles

Supported by the
American Academy of Ophthalmology

PREFACE

This report, prepared for the American Academy of Ophthalmology, examines the current and future requirements for eye care providers. It should be of interest to those who are interested in health care manpower issues and the interaction of manpower and health care systems.

The study estimates the supply, demand, and need for eye care providers: ophthalmologists, non-ophthalmic physicians, and optometrists. A typology of eye care services is developed which defines four domains of eye care: problem-oriented, rehabilitative, elective, and preventive eye care services. Requirements for services are determined in two ways: public health need and demand for eye care services. Public health need for eye care services is estimated using epidemiologically-determined population-based incidence and prevalence rates for individual eye diseases, and applying these rates to age-, gender-, and race-specific population estimates. Demand for eye care services is estimated using publicly available information from national utilization surveys that provide disease-specific use rates. Provider supply of ophthalmologists and optometrists is estimated from professional membership lists, American Medical Association information, and census information. We conducted a subspecialty-specific survey of practicing ophthalmologists to collect information on disease-specific treatment worktime requirements for medical and surgical eye care services. We reconcile need, demand, and supply using linear programming methods that allocate providers to disease groupings according to the provider type training requirements.

SUMMARY

INTRODUCTION

With the recent debate about health care reform, renewed interest has been engendered in workforce planning for health care in the United States. Whereas workforce issues once focused on a shortage of physicians and the geographic distribution of care, the discussion now focuses on a perceived surplus of physicians and the use of generalist versus specialist physicians, in part because specialist physicians are perceived to utilize more resources than generalists in the care of similar patients (Greenfield et al., 1992).

With this policy backdrop, the American Academy of Ophthalmology (AAO) commissioned RAND to conduct a workforce study of eye care providers and determine the requirements for eye care services in the United States. The three goals of the study were to: 1) quantify the supply of available providers of eye care; 2) estimate both the public health need and the current level of utilization (demand) for eye care services; and 3) reconcile the supply of providers with the demand and need for services to determine the extent of any imbalance that might exist.

The study explicitly encompasses the range of providers and services that constitute the eye care "market." Optometrists, comprehensive ophthalmologists, subspecialty ophthalmologists, and non-ophthalmologist physicians are all included as potential independent providers of eye care. Traditional physician services, such as problem- or disease-oriented acute and chronic care, are included; in addition, the study expands the universe of services to include rehabilitative (low vision), elective (cosmetic contacts and refractive surgery), and preventive services.

Consistent with other workforce studies, the current study does not address issues related to the quality or cost-effectiveness of care delivered under the various models. Instead services are analyzed according to what is legally allowed and no position is taken on the desirability of current work or care patterns. As additional data on quality, cost-effectiveness, and outcomes become available, this study, as well as other workforce studies, can be revised to incorporate these important data.

The study utilized a wide range of data sources, both primary and secondary. A primary data collection was undertaken through a survey of the practice and care patterns of ophthalmologists. The survey instruments and the collected data were reviewed by a multidisciplinary Advisory Panel, individual ophthalmologists and optometrists, and staff from the National Eye Institute.

Methods

To estimate the balance between workforce supply and requirements for eye care, three distinct models were used: the *supply* of eye care providers; the *public health need* for eye care; and the current *demand* for, or *utilization* of, eye care services. The supply model includes both ophthalmologists and optometrists (and non-ophthalmic physicians) as independent eye care providers. The *public health need* model employs epidemiological methods to determine the extent of eye disease in the population. The *demand* model uses nationally representative utilization data to determine the level of services currently used. The three models were organized to encompass those eye care services traditional to ophthalmic care patterns, organized into four domains of care: preventive, low vision / rehabilitation, elective, and problem-oriented. However, the study does not include vision training, eye muscle exercises, or other services that have traditionally been offered by optometrists, because information was not available on the extent of these services (the American Optometric Association (AOA) did not participate in the study).

The four domains of care were used to organize the available information related to the myriad of eye care services provided. Preventive care was defined to include primary prevention or well-eye examinations. Elective care was limited to cosmetic contact lenses and refractive surgery. Within the problem-oriented and low vision / rehabilitation domains, the thousands of codes in the *International*

Classification of Diseases, Revision 9 (ICD-9) and *Current Physician Procedure Terminology*, Revision 4 (CPT-4), were organized into 93 condition or disease groups and four low vision or rehabilitation groups. Each diagnostic code was assigned to one, and only one, condition group. These 93 condition groups, which formed the basis of the problem-oriented domain of care, were then re-aggregated into 14 condition categories. The four condition groups constituting the rehabilitative domain of eye care were re-aggregated into one condition category. Procedures were also assigned to condition groups and categories. However, since a given procedure might be used in the treatment of more than one condition, procedure codes were not uniquely assigned to a particular disease group. Instead, procedure codes were matched to diagnosis codes where clinically indicated. Finally, the groups and categories were organized to parallel accepted clinical distinctions and ophthalmology subspecialties.

To further organize the services that are provided, the study separated care into medical and surgical components. The medical component was separated into incident and prevalent cases to reflect the fact that new patients generally take longer to examine and treat or monitor than do continuing patients. The surgical component was subdivided into laser and incisional surgery. The surgical component, for both laser and incisional procedures, included the pre-operative assessment, the operative and same-day physician time, and the post-operative care in the first 90 days. This approach provided the framework for estimating the time required for care under the need and demand models.

The models use time as a common metric to measure supply, demand, and need. Work-time minutes was selected instead of patient encounters because future changes in care can be easily incorporated and work-time minutes are a more basic unit of measurement than number of encounters (i.e., all encounters can be translated into minutes while minutes cannot as easily be translated into number of encounters).

Workforce Requirements: Public Health Need

The *need* for eye care services is defined as the level of eye-related pathology in the population that requires monitoring or medical treatment. Thus, *need* includes not only those persons who are currently being treated (*demand*) but also those persons who have a given condition or disease and who might benefit from being seen by an eye care provider. As seen in Figure S.1, the need for eye care services for problem-oriented and low vision services was estimated using population-based incidence (new-patient) and prevalence (continuing-patient) rates. These rates were determined through several large, eye-oriented, epidemiological studies, such as Beaver Dam, Framingham, and Baltimore, which established the incidence and prevalence rates for many of the major eye conditions. In addition, Prevent Blindness America shared its rates for cataracts, glaucoma, diabetic retinopathy, visual impairment, and macular degeneration. Because rates do not exist for all eye conditions, condition-specific utilization information was used as a lower bound for incidence and prevalence for such conditions. Then, using the need-to-demand ratio for similar conditions for which incidence and prevalence information were available, the utilization-based demand information was adjusted upward to a number likely to be more reflective of need. The incidence and prevalence rates were then applied to Census Bureau estimates and projections of the United States population, disaggregated by demographic characteristics, such as age, gender, and race. The result from this calculation is the total number of persons who might need services for their eye condition.

However, not all patients with a given condition require monitoring on a schedule more frequent than what is accomplished through routine

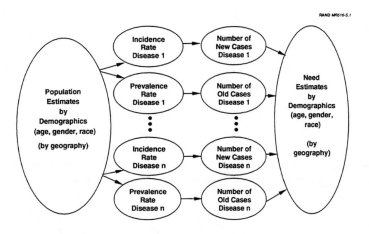

Fig. S.1--Estimation of Population Need for Eye Care Services

preventive or primary eye examination visits. As such, where data existed to provide estimates of the proportion of people who clinically need care, a downward adjustment to arrive at a "clinical population" was made. All such adjustments were reviewed by the Advisory Panel.

Estimates for the number of people needing preventive care were generated from application of the AAO's Preferred Practice Pattern on Comprehensive Adult Eye Examination (for adults) and the National Eye Care Forum (March 1994) schedule (for those younger than 18 years) to that proportion of the United States population that did not require problem-oriented or low vision care. Patients receiving problem-oriented or low vision care are assumed to receive the needed primary eye care services during their visits. Estimates for elective services were derived from anecdotal evidence, further adjusted by the expert judgement of the Advisory Panel. Once the number of people needing care was determined, the care needed for each individual (described below in a later section) was applied and the results aggregated to a total number of minutes of care needed.

Demand or Utilization

Demand for eye care services was estimated using publicly available national utilization surveys. For preventive services, the model used the current level of preventive visits for *demand* as opposed to the recommended Preferred Practice Pattern and National Eye Care Forum schedules for need (Bennett and Aron, 1993). Two data sets were particularly useful: the National Ambulatory Medical Care Survey (NAMCS) and the National Hospital Discharge Survey (NHDS). These surveys include diagnostic and procedure information for doctor office visits and hospitalizations, respectively. Certain ambulatory settings are excluded from the NAMCS, such as hospital-based clinics (which exclude many clinics in academic medical centers), Veterans Administration facilities, emergency rooms, and others. However, these excluded sites account for less than six percent of the overall utilization of eye care services (Lewin, 1992). From these data, condition-specific utilization was calculated, which when applied to national population estimates, resulted in the demand estimates (see Figure S.2).

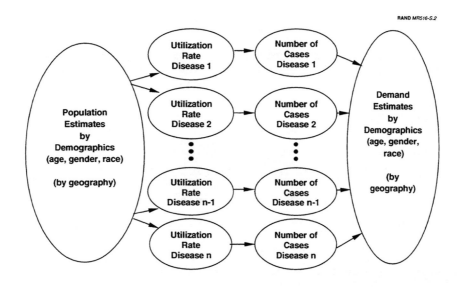

RAND MR516-S.2

Fig. S.2--Estimation of Population Demand for Eye Care Services

The Medicare Part B files provided additional data for comparison to the model's demand predictions for those conditions most frequently occurring in the elderly population. In only five of 93 condition groups, representing less than one percent of the total volume of services, were discrepancies found; the predicted utilization was then adjusted upwards to reflect the higher utilization reported in the Part B data.

Using information from the NAMCS, the condition-specific number of persons demanding care was adjusted downward by the average number of eye conditions per person being reported out of an ophthalmologist's office. The visit time was then adjusted to reflect the marginal time required to care for a patient with multiple conditions, using the length of visits for the NAMCS averages for patients with one, two, or three or more conditions (with one condition being a base time of one and multiple conditions being fractionally larger then one). This adjustment was made to reflect that the time to treat multiple conditions was less than the sum of the times to treat the individual conditions. These adjustments were also applied to the public health need estimates.

Supply of Eye Care Providers

The total supply of eye care providers includes ophthalmologists, other physicians, and optometrists. To simplify the analysis, the current level of care provided by other (non-ophthalmologist) physicians was continued throughout the analysis. The remaining services provided by ophthalmologists and optometrists were the focus of the modeling. The membership file of the AAO was used to quantify the number of ophthalmologists in the United States. This file consists of information on all ophthalmologists, members and nonmembers of the AAO, including information on board certification, self-identified ophthalmic subspecialty, and certain demographic characteristics, such as age and gender. These data were compared with Census Bureau data and were found to be quantitatively similar, and richer in demographic and training information. Data for optometrists was more difficult to obtain because the American Optometric Association declined to participate in the study. Data from numerous sources were examined, and those from the 1990 census Public Use Microdata Sample, which provided occupation (i.e., optometrist) as well as minimal demographic information (i.e., age, gender, and state of residence), were used. The estimates derived from the Census Bureau files were very similar to the total number of active optometrists estimated by the AOA.

The supply model determined the current number of ophthalmologists and optometrists in practice, as well as estimated the inflow and the outflow of providers. The inflow consists of new trainees entering into the supply pool; the outflow consists of those persons exiting the supply pool due to retirement and death. For the optometric supply projections, it is assumed that all new optometrists will be trained for therapeutic drug privileges. Figure S.3 illustrates the components on the supply model.

The study used the concept of full-time equivalent (FTE) as the metric for counting providers. An *FTE* is defined by the total number of hours, per year, in which eye care services can be provided and is a function of the number of hours worked per day and the number of weeks worked per year. According to the American Medical Association's annual survey of physicians, which includes a sample of ophthalmologists,

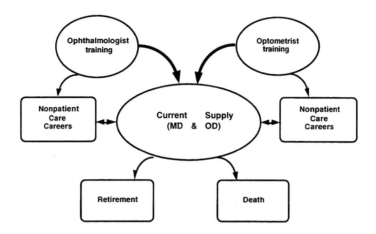

Fig. S.3--Provider Supply Model

ophthalmologists, on average, spend 42 hours per week in direct patient care activities, 48 weeks per year. Thus, an FTE was defined as providing 2,016 hours of patient care work each year. The FTE is an unit of analysis for workforce planning and carries no implications of quality or cost-effectiveness. *Direct patient care activities* are those activities that would hold regardless of the financing or delivery system. As such, they include not only the diagnosis and treatment of the patient but also the time required for reviewing the chart, discussing the diagnosis and treatment options with the patient and family, and documenting in the chart. Not included in this time, however, are those activities that relate to practice-specific or payor-specific paperwork requirements.

In relating FTEs to individual providers, certain adjustments were made. First, providers in training were given only a fraction of the work time available to reflect their lower productivity (time and efficiency) in seeing patients (0.35 FTE in the first clinical year, 0.5 FTE in each of the following years). Second, an adjustment was made for gender (0.85 FTE for women), in line with accepted workforce methods (Schwartz, Sloan, and Mendelson, 1988). Third, full-time academic ophthalmologists were estimated at 0.5 FTE for patient care activities, in recognition of their other activities, such as research, teaching, and administration.

Disease- and Procedure-Specific Work-Time Estimates

For this workforce analysis, the companion information to the incidence and prevalence information is the amount of labor input required to treat persons with particular eye conditions. Such information is not available in the literature for the vast majority of conditions and services. Consequently, a survey of 2,007 ophthalmologists practicing in the United States was conducted to determine the amount of time required to treat patients medically and surgically for specific eye conditions. Because the American Optometric Association did not participate in the study, a parallel survey of optometrists was not conducted. Instead, a work-time ratio was used to reflect the potential differential amount of time optometrists require to provide eye care services compared to ophthalmologists for those conditions that optometrists are legally allowed to provide medical care. Because anecdotal evidence and optometric trade journals suggest that the number of hours worked each year by the average optometrist may be less than that of an average ophthalmologist, and that the amount of time used by optometrists in caring for patients may be longer, a range of work-time ratios between 0.6 and 1 was used and workforce estimates provided for each ratio. The work-time ratio of 1 reflects the null hypothesis that both types of providers supply the same level of patient care time and use the same amount of time to care for similar patients. A work-time ratio of 0.6 reflects an alternative hypothesis that optometrists supply fewer patient care hours, use some available time to provide services not included in this study, and/or take more time in the care of patients. The work-time ratio does not imply differences or equivalencies in the quality or cost-effectiveness of care; it is an analytical device used to overcome the lack of data concerning optometric-specific work times. In addition, the work-time ratio is a way to incorporate the impact of optometric services that have not been included explicitly in this study.

Ophthalmic subspecialty-specific surveys were developed for the nine major ophthalmic subspecialties (Cataract, Cornea, Glaucoma, Low Vision, Neuro Ophthalmology, Pediatrics and Strabismus, Plastics and Reconstructive, Retina, and Uveitis) that could be identified in the AAO membership files and for General Ophthalmology. Each survey includes diagnoses and procedures particular to each subspecialty; the subspecialty-specific lists of diagnoses and procedures were developed with consultation from the various subspecialty organizations.

The survey had five major sections: (1) practice-specific characteristics; (2) work-time requirements for the initial medical visits for patients with certain diagnoses; (3) work-time requirements for follow-up medical care for the same diagnosis; (4) the percentage of patients having the same diagnosis who proceed to surgery (incisional or laser) each year; and (5) work-time requirements for the pre-operative, post-operative, and intra-operative period for a specified list of procedures. In addition, ample space was provided for additional diagnoses or procedures to be added if the respondent desired; fewer than one percent of respondents did so.

The response rate for the survey was 40 percent, which provided sufficient data to develop statistically stable work-time estimates. Using the survey data, work times were calculated for the medical and surgical components of care for the diagnoses and procedures used in the study.

Reconciliation of Care Requirements and Provider Supply

The public health need for eye care service was obtained by multiplying the time required to provide care by the number of individuals in the "clinical population" in each of the 97 condition groups, elective care, and preventive care. The available work time supply was calculated by aggregating across FTEs by provider type. The total number of patient care minutes required (by need or demand) was divided by the available FTEs to yield the number of such providers needed. These calculations generated providers required by condition group, provider type, or subspecialty area.

Once the supply of providers of eye care and the need and demand for eye care services are known, workforce planning entails a reconciliation of supply with requirements. From this reconciliation, it is possible to make judgments concerning the undersupply or oversupply of providers to satisfy need and/or demand. The reconciliation takes place using condition-specific minutes of care *supplied* by types of care (that is, medical or surgical) and allocating the time to *need* or *demand* determined condition-specific numbers of patients. The process of reconciliation also highlights the various assumptions made in the three models and provides an opportunity to examine the robustness of the results under different assumptions.

Because the reconciliation process required assumptions to be made about the structure of the health care system, the study posited three different health care delivery system scenarios that define how patients initially access providers: optometrists first, ophthalmologists first, and a primary care provider model where optometrists and general ophthalmologists share primary care service provision. Services needed or demanded are first allocated to those providers who can perform such services; once those providers are exhausted or services they cannot provide remain, those services are allocated to the other provider type. The models are described as follows:

- The *optometrist-first* model allocates patients first to optometrists with diagnostic drug privileges (DPA) and then to optometrists with therapeutic drug privileges (TPA). When the optometric provider supply is exhausted or services are required which cannot be provided by optometrists, patients are allocated to ophthalmologists. The allocation between optometrists can be easily adjusted because TPA optometrists can displace DPA optometrists, but not always vice versa. Similarly, ophthalmologists can displace optometrists, but not necessarily vice versa.

- The *ophthalmologist-first* model allocates patients to general ophthalmologists first, then to subspecialty ophthalmologists, and finally to optometrists, with priority in allocation to ophthalmologists for those services that only ophthalmologists can perform.

- The *primary care provider* model allocates patients to optometrists and general ophthalmologists initially, and then to subspecialist ophthalmologists if any patients remain.

These three delivery system scenarios provide a range of options in which ophthalmologists and optometrists are providers of care. None of the models reflect the current delivery system, which includes many variants on these themes. However, these scenarios define system boundaries, establishing limits to the estimates of surplus or shortage by provider type. The allocation of patients to providers in the reconciliation is accomplished through linear programming using a scoring system that assigns priority to provider types for allocation to need and demand categories.

In view of concern about the enormous number of variables included in the models of this study and the use of data from disparate sources (i.e., different samples and surveys), the study examined the effect of data variation and possible sample error on the stability of the final results. First, the study used the bootstrap, a statistical technique that resamples the data from surveys or population samples (with replacement) so that the model's calculations can be repeated and the results compared (Efron and Tibshirani, 1993). From the bootstrap, the distribution of possible results emerges, yielding a plausible range of results or area of confidence. Second, the models and reconciliation were examined for statistical robustness. Random statistical variation was introduced into the data and the models were run and the results compared. Thus, all of the components in the models were "shaken up" by sizable amounts and the random variations were then carried through to the final calculations. The distribution of results revealed a short confidence interval around the final results, indicating that adjustments to any given data variable are unlikely to significantly alter the overall results.

RESULTS

The results of the workforce analysis show that, overall, there is a large surplus of eye care providers in the United States (Table S.1). However, the characteristics of the surplus vary according to the health care delivery system posited (Table S.2).

Table S.1 shows the current demand and need for eye care providers relative to supply. The total FTE supply of providers decreases as the work-time ratios for optometrists decrease. No matter what type of health care delivery system is postulated, the estimated need and demand for services is constant because the same work times and FTE definitions are used. Thus, there is a current requirement of 30,757 FTE eye care providers to satisfy the population's need for services, and a requirement of 22,154 FTE eye care providers to satisfy the population's demand for services. The simple comparison of supply and demand or need shows that a surplus exists relative to demand across the range of work-time ratios for optometrists. This surplus is robust to the data, with a standard error of about 2,000 FTEs.

Table S.1
Demand and Need for Eye Care Services Relative to Supply

Work-Time Ratios	Number of FTE Optometrists	Number of FTE Ophthalmologists	Total FTE Supply	FTEs Demanded	FTEs Needed
1.0	27,646	14,091	41,737	22,154	30,757
0.8	22,117	14,091	36,208	22,154	30,757
0.6	16,588	14,091	30,679	22,154	30,757

Table S.2 presents the results of reconciliation when public health need is allocated to optometrist or ophthalmologist providers under the two extreme boundary scenarios: optometrists first and ophthalmologists first. As stated above, a range of estimates was calculated, reflecting different work-time ratios for optometrists. The results indicate that ophthalmologists would be in surplus in the optometry-first model. Optometrists, on the other hand, are in surplus, except when the work-time ratio is 0.6 or less in the ophthalmologist-first model or when the work-time ratio is 0.8 or less in the optometry-first model. Again,

these results highlight the need for additional data to better
understand optometric care patterns and to determine the appropriate
work-time ratio.

Table S.2
Allocation of Care Under Two Delivery-System Scenarios,
Public Health Need

Type of Provider and Work-Time Ratios	Supply	Optometry First		Ophthalmology First	
		Required	Excess	Required	Excess
Ophthalmology	14,091	7,800	6,291	14,091	0
Optometry					
1.0	27,646	22,957	4,689	16,666	10,980
0.8	22,117	22,957	0	16,666	5,451
0.6	16,588	22,957	0	16,666	0

NOTE: Under a 0.6 work-time ratio for the optometrist-first model, the
net effect is to eliminate the ophthalmologist surplus.

In addition, the influence of a number of factors on the overall
results was examined. For example, it could be postulated that the age
of the ophthalmologist or provider may affect the work times reported.
However, when "old" versus "young" ophthalmologist work times and care
patterns were compared through the full reconciliation model, there was
less than a five percent difference in estimating need, with older
providers exhibiting shorter work times. Thus, no separate adjustment
was made for provider age. Other factors that were examined include
region of the country and practice structure (i.e., the number of
clinical assistants used in the practice). Neither of these factors
significantly changed the overall results.

Of note, the number of patient visits for preventive care, and thus
the time needed to provide such care, is *higher* under the demand model
than under the need model, because current utilization for such visits
exceeds that recommended by the Preferred Practice Pattern and the
National Eye Care Forum. The AOA estimates that nearly 78 million
primary eye examinations were performed (Bennett and Aron, 1993), as

opposed to the 45 million that would be called for under the National Eye Care Forum proposed schedule and the 59 million under the Preferred Practice Pattern (adults) and National Eye Care Forum (pediatric age) schedules used in the need model. However, current utilization levels are lower than would be predicted under the proposed preventive visit schedule of the AOA.

FUTURE PROJECTIONS

The requirements for satisfying need for eye care services were projected into the future, to years 2000 and 2010, using a workforce supply projection that assumed training of ophthalmologists and optometrists would remain at the current level and that distribution of subspecialization remains constant. Need was estimated using the same incidence and prevalence rates applied to future population projections disaggregated by age, gender, and race. As with the analysis of the current workforce reconciliation of requirements to supply, there is an excess of eye care providers, even though the need for services is increased because of a projected larger and older population.

DISCUSSION

The model results in this study clearly indicate that a sizable surplus of eye care providers exists relative to current utilization patterns or demand within the range of work-time ratios used in this study. This finding is consistent with those of other reports. First, a 1990 survey of ophthalmologists reported in *Medical Economics* revealed that 49 percent believed they were practicing below capacity (Clark, 1990). Second, the demand for approximately 9,000 problem-oriented care providers practicing 2,016 hours per year is similar to the projections of eye care workforce needs that result from applying staff model HMO ratios of ophthalmologists to enrollees. An HMO ophthalmologists-to-enrollee ratio of 3:100,000 applied to the national population of over 250 million persons yields a demand for 7,500 full-time ophthalmologists (Weiner, 1994).

Third, many staff model HMOs employ two optometrists to every one ophthalmologist. Using this ratio, roughly 15,000 optometrists would be employed for every 7,500 ophthalmologists. This supports the study's findings that there is a surplus of providers. Relative to the current demand of 22,154 total providers predicted by the model using the care patterns of ophthalmologists (and a work-time ratio of 1), the total of 22,500 providers demanded under an HMO staffing model is quite comparable. Because the HMO staffing ratios explored by Weiner come from staff model HMOs and not from capitated group practice IPA models, applying Weiner's adjustment for the presence of group IPA models still results in a surplus of providers.

The conclusions are generally similar when public health need is examined. Thus, even if health care reform were to increase access to eye care services for every person, there would *still* be an excess of providers, unless the work-time ratio for optometrists is 0.6 or less. Given the fact that even under free universal care there would be a segment of the population that would not use care for other reasons, the surplus of providers would be even larger. Such a conclusion, however, is based on the care patterns currently being used. If utilization were to involve an increase in the intensity of services by 40 percent, then equilibrium could be approached, even with a work-time ratio of 1. Given that the need model assumes that care patterns today represent appropriate care, significant new data indicating the value of more visits, or more extensive visits, would have to be presented to support such an increase in service intensity.

Concerns about the validity of the data elements used in creating the care patterns assumed in the current study can be addressed, although not completely alleviated, in the absence of large-scale time-motion studies or work-journal methods. As discussed in the Methods section, numerous statistical techniques were used to test the robustness of the results. This process and the generation of the range of possible values, and the review of individual data elements by ophthalmologists, optometrists, and an expert advisory panel all engender a high degree of confidence in the basic direction of the conclusions.

FUTURE RESEARCH

The questions of whether or which provider types--ophthalmologists, optometrists, and other physicians--should be reduced were beyond the scope of this project. There are no scientifically determined data on quality of care, patient outcomes, costs, and cost-effectiveness for comparable patients treated by different provider types. The ability to answer these questions could be inferred from training background, education, and other factors, but such inferences are guesses and are not based on scientifically derived standards. Thus, data on how optometrists deliver care, how integrated delivery systems deliver care, how care patterns can potentiate or detract from desirable outcomes, and other similar questions are central to providing information to more rational workforce planning. This is a limitation faced by *all* workforce planning efforts and is not unique to this study, or eye care services. The need for data is perhaps the central challenge facing workforce planning. As more data become available, health policy analysts can embark on more refined and accurate projections of workforce supply and requirements, and more accurately model the dynamic nature of health care and the care of patients. By incorporating knowledge of the outcomes and the cost-effectiveness of care, workforce planning can begin to help contribute to optimizing the delivery of health care.

ACKNOWLEDGMENTS

This report benefitted from the comments and suggests of various members of the ophthalmology community. We gratefully acknowledge the members of the ophthalmic subspecialty organizations (John Hunkeler, M.D. (Cataract), James McCulley, M.D. (Cornea), Allan Kolker, M.D. (Glaucoma), Michael Fischer, M.D. (low vision), David Guyton, M.D., and Walter Fierson, M.D. (Pediatrics and Strabismus), Albert Hornblass, M.D. (Plastics), James Sharpe, M.D. (Neuro-ophthalmology), Harry Flynn, M.D., and J. Wallace McMeel, M.D. (Retina), Ira Wong, M.D. (Uveitis), Richard Lindstrom, M.D. (refractive surgery), and Melvin Freeman, M.D. (Contact Lens) and the members of our Advisory Panel (Wayne Bizer, D.O., Bernice Brown, M.D., Neil Choplin, M.D., Walter Fierson, M.D., Melvin Freeman, M.D., Kevin Greenidge, M.D., Steve Kamenetzky, M.D., Carol Mangione, M.D., James McCulley, M.D., Joel Sacks, M.D., James Salz, M.D., John Shepherd, M.D., Robert Stamper, M.D., Allen Verne, M.D., Ira Wong, M.D., and Mark Wood, M.D.) for their helpful suggestions and comments. We would also like to thank Leon Elwein, M.D., and Valeria Friedlin from The National Eye Institute, Ms. Sherry Delio from Virginia Mason Medical Center, and Rohit Varma, M.D., and John Michon, M.D., from the University of Southern California for data contributions and discussions. In addition, we would like to thank Prevent Blindness America and James Tielsch, Ph.D., for sharing incidence and prevalence rate data with this study.

Finally, we would like to thank Jonathan Weiner, Dr.P.H., from The Johns Hopkins University and Emmett Keeler, Ph.D., from RAND for their review and insightful comments on the report.

We would also like to thank our RAND colleagues. Marian Branch provided expert editorial guidance, helping us to organize the report and to improve the clarity of our writing. Joan Buchanan, Ph.D., Susan Hosek, M.S., Arleen Leibowitz, Ph.D., and Emmett Keeler, Ph.D., provided very helpful comments and suggestions at the start of the study. Carol Mangione, M.D., provided helpful comments throughout the project. Marygail Brauner, Ph.D., helped us in formulating and solving our linear

programming approach to reconciling requirements with supply. Julie
Brown provided expert assistance in the conduct of the survey. Dee
Hutchison and Helen Rhodes provided secretarial and administrative
support to the project.

CONTENTS

PREFACE... iii

SUMMARY.. iv
   INTRODUCTION.. iv
      Methods v
      Workforce Requirements: Public Health Need vi
      Demand or Utilization viii
      Supply of Eye Care Providers x
      Disease- and Procedure-Specific Work-Time Estimates xii
      Reconciliation of Care Requirements and Provider Supply .. xiii
   RESULTS.. xvi
   FUTURE PROJECTIONS..................................... xviii
   DISCUSSION... xviii
   FUTURE RESEARCH.. xx

ACKNOWLEDGMENTS... xxi

FIGURES.. xxvi

TABLES.. xxvii

Chapter

1. INTRODUCTION.. 1
   REVIEW OF PRIOR MEDICAL WORKFORCE ANALYSES.................... 2
      Graduate Medical Education National Advisory Committee 3
      American Academy of Ophthalmology (AAO) 4
      Bureau of Health Professions (BHPr) 4
      American Medical Association 5
      Population-to-Workforce Ratio Studies 6
   ANALYSIS OF APPROACHES..................................... 7
   CURRENT ISSUES.. 8
   SUMMARY.. 11

2. THE MODEL: ISSUES AND CONCEPTUAL FRAMEWORK...................... 12
   INTRODUCTION... 12
   DOMAINS OF EYE CARE SERVICES.............................. 13
   STEP 1. ORGANIZE DIAGNOSIS AND PROCEDURE CODES BY DOMAINS OF
       CARE 14
   STEP 2. SURVEY AVAILABLE DATA............................. 19
      Supply 19
      Demand 21
      Need 23
   STEP 3. ESTABLISH POPULATION PREVALENCE, INCIDENCE, AND
       CLINICAL RATES 27
      Need--Prevalence and Incidence Rates 27
      Need--Determination of Clinical Rates 29
      Demand--Old and New Visit Rates 31
      Preventive and Elective Rates 32

STEP 4. CONDUCT SURVEY OF WORKTIMES AND CLINICAL CARE·
    REQUIREMENTS 32
STEP 5. CALCULATE AVAILABLE FTE PROVIDERS.................... 34
STEP 6. CALCULATE FTE REQUIREMENTS AND RECONCILE WITH FTE
    SUPPLY 36
STEP 7. ADDRESS DATA LIMITATIONS AND DATA VARIATIONS......... 38
    Limitations of the Data 38
    Methods for Addressing Data Limitations 39
STEP 8. FUTURE PROJECTION.................................... 40
SUMMARY.. 40

3. SUPPLY OF EYE CARE PROVIDERS.................................... 42
    SUPPLY OF OPHTHALMOLOGISTS.................................. 42
    Number of Ophthalmologists 42
    Residents and Fellows in Training 43
    Adjustments to the Number of Ophthalmologists 45
    Projecting the Supply of Ophthalmologists 46
    Work-Time Estimates 47
    SUPPLY OF OPTOMETRISTS...................................... 48
    Number of Optometrists 49
    Inflow 52
    Outflow 53
    Capacity 54
    Final Assumptions 55
    Projecting the Supply of Optometrists 58
    OTHER PHYSICIAN SUPPLY..................................... 59
    SUMMARY.. 61

4. NEED AND DEMAND FOR EYE CARE PROVIDERS........................ 62
    CLINICAL NEED... 63
    PROVIDER WORK TIMES.. 64
    Office Visit Times 64
    Surgery Times (Laser and Incisional) 67
    Survey Data Time Estimates 67
    NEED AND DEMAND SPREADSHEET COMPUTATIONS.................... 73
    Differences in Computing Need Versus Demand 74
    Office Work Computations 76
    Surgical Work Computations 77
    Preventive Services 78
    Elective Services 79
    Spreadsheet Computation Results 80
    Summary 80

5. SUPPLY AND REQUIREMENTS RECONCILIATION........................ 82
    RECONCILIATION METHODS..................................... 82
    Problem Setup 82
    Reconciliation Results 86
    ROBUSTNESS OF THE RESULTS.................................. 92
    Accounting for Uncertainty 92
    Optometrist / Ophthalmologist Work-Time Ratios 93
    RAND Eye Care Workforce Survey: Response Bias Effects 95
    Stability Across Census Regions 96
    SUMMARY.. 98

6. CONCLUSIONS AND POLICY IMPLICATIONS............................. 99
    EXCESS RELATIVE TO DELIVERY SYSTEM............................ 99
        Comprehensive Ophthalmology 100
        Relative Quality of Care Provided 101
        Demand and the Surplus 101
        Summary 102
    STRUCTURAL DECISIONS AND ALTERNATIVE MODELS.................. 103
        Number of Work Hours per Year 103
        Provider-Type Differences 104
        Preventive Services Package 105
        Conceptual Framework 106
        Health Care Structure and Financing: Work Hour Changes ... 106
        Other Influences on Workforce Size 107
        Need and Surplus 108
    COMPARISON TO OTHER WORKFORCE METHODOLOGIES................. 108
    POLICY IMPLICATIONS.. 110

Appendix A   METHODS USED TO GROUP DIAGNOSES AND PROCEDURES CREATING
    THE 97 DISEASE GROUPS AND THE 15 DISEASE CATEGORIES 113
    CREATION OF THE LIST OF DIAGNOSES.......................... 113
    CREATION OF LIST OF PROCEDURES AND SERVICES................ 115
    LINKAGE OF DISEASES AND PROCEDURES AND SERVICES............ 117
    SUMMARY.. 118
Appendix B   WORK TIME AND REQUIREMENTS ESTIMATES.................. 119

REFERENCES.. 132

FIGURES

Fig. S.1-Estimation of Population Need for Eye Care Services....... vii

Fig. S.2-Estimation of Population Demand for Eye Care Services...... ix

Fig. S.3-Provider Supply Model.................................... xi

Fig. 2.1-Domains of Eye Care Services, With Disease Groups and
      Categories 15

Fig. 2.2-Estimation of Population Need for Eye Care Services........ 31

Fig. 2.3-Estimation of Population Demand for Eye Care Services...... 32

Fig. 2.4-RAND Survey of Ophthalmologist Practice Patterns
      (sample page) 35

Fig. 2.5-Provider Supply Model..................................... 36

Fig. 4.1-RAND Eye Care Workforce Survey: Initial Medical Visits.... 65

Fig. 4.2-RAND Eye Care Workforce Survey: Follow-up Visits.......... 66

Fig. 4.3-RAND Eye Care Workforce Survey: Pre-Operative Assessment
      and Intra-Operative Time 68

Fig. 4.4-RAND Eye Care Workforce Survey: Post-Operative Period..... 69

TABLES

Table S.1 Demand and Need for Eye Care Services Relative to Supply xvi

Table S.2 Allocation of Care Under Two Delivery-System Scenarios, Public Health Need xvii

Table 2.1 Problem-Oriented and Rehabilitative Categories and Groupings of Care 15

Table 2.2 Data for Supply Estimation............................. 20

Table 2.3 Data for Demand Estimation............................ 22

Table 2.4 Data for Need Estimation.............................. 24

Table 2.5 National Eye Care Forum Preventive Eye Care Services Schedule 26

Table 2.6 Source of Incidence and Prevalence (Need) Information by Disease Category 30

Table 3.1 Number of Active Ophthalmologists (members and fellows), by Subspecialty: 1994 43

Table 3.2 Distribution of Fellows, by Subspecialty: 1994.......... 44

Table 3.3 Projected Number of Ophthalmologists: 1994-2010........ 46

Table 3.4 AMA Work Time Data: FTE Definition.................... 48

Table 3.5 Distribution of Optometrists by State and Type of Privileges 50

Table 3.6 1992-1993 U.S. Optometry School Graduates by Race and Gender 53

Table 3.7 Types of Diseases Treated by Optometrists, by Disease Group 57

Table 3.8 Projected Number of Optometrists: 1994-2010............. 58

Table 3.9 Proportion of Eye Care Diseases Treated by Non-Ophthalmologist Physicians, By Disease Group 60

Table 4.1 Components of Office Work Time......................... 71

Table 4.2 Components of Incisional and Laser Surgical Times........ 72

Table 4.3 Variables For Need and Demand Spreadsheet Computations... 73

Table 4.4 Final Estimates of Demand and Need from Spreadsheet...... 80

Table 5.1 Format of Data Table for Reconciliation Step............. 83

Table 5.2 Assignments of Multipliers for the Linear Programming
    Algorithm 87

Table 5.3 Summary Description of Supply, Requirements, and Excesses, by
    Model, Type of Provider, and Year 88

Table 5.4 Assignments from Linear Programming, Optometry-First
    Structure 90

Table 5.5 Demand and Need for Eye Care Services Relative to Supply. 94

Table 5.6 Allocation of Care Under Two Delivery-System Scenarios,
    Public Health Need 95

Table 5.7 Comparison of Full Survey Population with Responding Survey
    Population 97

Table 5.8 Distribution of Reconciliation Across Census Regions..... 98

Table B.1 Components of Office Work Time........................ 120

Table B.2 Components of Incisional and Laser Surgical Times....... 123

Table B.3 Final Estimates of Demand and Need from Spreadsheet..... 129

1. INTRODUCTION

The size and composition of the medical workforce have been public policy concerns since the early 1900s. Policymakers and the medical profession want to assure themselves and the public that there will be a sufficient supply of well-trained medical professionals. This was the motivation, in part, for the Flexner Report (Flexner, 1910) at the turn of the century, which revolutionized how physicians were trained in the United States. As medicine has become more specialized, issues surrounding medical education and workforce characteristics have become more complex. Today, policymakers are still concerned about the numbers of professionals, but they are also increasingly concerned with the specialty distribution. Evidence to date has suggested that the specialization of medicine has contributed to increased health care costs (Greenfield et al., 1992). In the absence of similar data on quality, policymakers are concerned that there may be too many specialist medical professionals and that this surplus may unnecessarily increase health care costs. In an environment of health care cost containment and reform, this concern is particularly acute (Mullan et al., 1993).

As health care reform is debated, it is an opportune time to revisit the issue of the *supply*--number of providers--and *requirements*--defined either as the economic demand for and actual utilization of services or the public health need for and the optimal level of utilization of services. The most cited effort to address health care workforce needs is the Graduate Medical Education National Advisory Committee (GMENAC) study, in 1981. The approach to medical workforce estimation pioneered by that study has formed the foundation of many subsequent analyses. The Bureau of Health Professions (BHPr) and the American Medical Association (AMA) have ongoing workforce projects, and other projections have been done by the Council on Graduate Medical Education (COGME) and the Physician Payment Review Commission (PPRC). However, the explosion of knowledge and technology in medicine over the

past decade and significant changes in insurance and financing have
altered some of the parameters under which such studies were conducted.

The American Academy of Ophthalmology (AAO) commissioned RAND to
conduct a study of the current and future supply, demand, and need for
eye care professionals. As with medicine in general, the practice of
ophthalmology has changed significantly over the past decade as
technical innovations have produced new procedures and refined old
procedures. Certain of these changes have increased productivity
tremendously. Moreover, the provision of eye care services has evolved
to include numerous professionals, including ophthalmologists, other
physicians, optometrists, and ophthalmic nurses, technicians, and
assistants. Indeed, all states permit optometrists to prescribe and use
diagnostic drugs, and 40 states allow optometrists to prescribe certain
therapeutic drugs. This wide array of eye care professionals means that
any study of the current and future supply, need, and demand for eye
care services must cover many participants of different disciplines and
varying levels of skill and experience.

REVIEW OF PRIOR MEDICAL WORKFORCE ANALYSES

Traditional estimations of workforce need and demand utilize one of
four approaches: workforce-to-population ratios; service targets;
health needs; and economic demand. The Department of Health, Education,
and Welfare in 1976 published a two-volume report reviewing these
approaches and their strengths and weaknesses (Kriesberg et al., 1976a,
1976b). What all approaches share is a distinction between the *supply*
of providers and the *requirements* for service. Thus, estimates of
workforce requirements must project, consolidate, and synthesize at
least two (supply and requirements) and possibly three (supply, demand,
and need) models.

Four prominent medical workforce studies conducted in recent years
are useful to describe and review in greater detail for the strengths
and weaknesses of their approaches. These are the 1981 GMENAC study,
the ongoing studies of the BHPr and the AMA, and the AAO's own 1978–1984
ophthalmology workforce study, which provides an alternative to the
preceding three broader-based studies. Recently, these and other

studies have been the focus of debate concerning what assumptions medical workforce studies should use (Singer 1989; Feil et al., 1993; Reuben et al., 1993; Rivo et al., 1993). Finally, several studies have been published recently using managed care systems' physician-to-population ratios to assess the number of physicians (generalists and specialists) required.

Graduate Medical Education National Advisory Committee

The extensive analysis of future U.S. physician workforce requirements conducted by GMENAC (1981) based physician supply estimates on the then current supply of physicians; the flow of students into medical school through residency programs; the flow of foreign medical students and foreign medical graduates (FMGs) into the domestic physician supply; and physician attrition due to death, retirement, and other reasons. Physician requirements were calculated on an adjusted needs-based approach, which modified public health need estimates of disease *incidence* (new) and *prevalence* (continuing) by utilization based on consumer demand patterns. Public health need was then adjusted to include the actual service requirements according to then current norms of care, which were ultimately adjusted by physician productivity estimates. The workforce estimates included non-patient-care activity time, such as that devoted to teaching, research, and administration. Although still controversial, the GMENAC results showed a surplus of 69,750 physicians overall, with particular surpluses and deficits by specialty. For ophthalmology, the GMENAC study estimated a total supply of 16,300 and a total need of 11,600, resulting in a surplus of 4,700 by the year 1990.

The GMENAC study used an approach that relied heavily on data from specialty-specific, multidisciplinary advisory panels. Those panels gathered material from divergent sources to understand and characterize the type of practice and the work efforts required for specific physician specialties. For ophthalmology, the panel acknowledged the contribution of optometrists in providing routine eye examinations and included them in its workforce estimates. The panel incorporated information on incidence and prevalence for a limited number of conditions or diseases into the need dimension of its estimates (which were based on 10 specific diagnosis codes, each accounting for 3 percent or more of the 1980 ophthalmology workload). Workforce calculations were based on a model comparing supply with adjusted need for services.

American Academy of Ophthalmology (AAO)

In contrast to the GMENAC report, the AAO report on ophthalmic workforce requirements projected a shortage of 3,000 ophthalmologists by the year 2000 (Ruiz, 1984). This report used the data from the GMENAC study and provided a reinterpretation, basing workforce requirements on a needs approach: the workforce that would be required if everyone who wanted an eye examination by an ophthalmologist was able to have one within a reasonable amount of time (e.g., 30 days) and if all ocular diseases were treated by physicians. The difference between the GMENAC and AAO findings results largely from the AAO's use of a greater number of visits to treat diabetic retinopathy and a doubling of the average length of time for office visits (Ruiz, 1984). In a series of papers, the AAO additionally published the results of its work on estimating the need for services (Reinecke, 1978); estimating the demand for eye care on the basis of public survey data (Reinecke and Steinberg, 1981); surveying the practice activity of 1,258 ophthalmologists in a variety of settings (Worthen et al., 1981); and studying the geographic distribution of ophthalmologists (Gamble et al., 1983).

It is useful to characterize the AAO workforce study as a reassessment of workforce requirements projected by the GMENAC study because it contributes to the debate on what assumptions should be used in such an analysis. It presents one end of workforce requirements estimates: meeting *all* the eye care services needed rather than accounting just for the amount of care demanded.

Bureau of Health Professions (BHPr)

The BHPr developed and currently maintains a model to forecast the nation's supply of physicians in the aggregate, by specialty, and by professional activity (Kindig et al., 1993). The model is composed of five separate models that interface with one another and share data elements. The supply models are (1) an aggregate model, (2) a specialty model, (3) a subnational allopathic model, (4) a subnational osteopathic model, and (5) a specialty distribution model. The BHPr model projects that there will be 17,845 ophthalmologists in the year 2000, and 20,459 in the year 2020 (Greenberg, 1992; Lewin, 1992).

A companion model forecasts the requirements for physicians by specialty, estimating the demand for physician services by type of service (e.g., doctor office visits, surgeries, etc.) and by patient characteristics such as age, race, and sex. These requirements are then converted into minutes-based physician requirements. AMA survey information on available physician time is used to calculate estimates of physician productivity and supply. The supply of physicians (converted into available provider minutes) is compared with the minutes-based requirements to yield estimates of surplus and deficit.

The BHPr model is a complex array of matrices describing the supply and demand for services. These matrices are related through straightforward relationships, such as the total supply of physician services, the weeks worked, and the hours worked per week. They fully characterize the supply and demand for services. Implicit in the characterization is a continuation of current utilization and productivity patterns into the future. In addition, only physician (M.D.) providers are considered.

American Medical Association

The AMA published its physician workforce study, *Physician Supply and Utilization by Specialty: Trends and Projections,* in 1988. This study gives a detailed estimate of the future supply of physicians and utilization trends for 13 different medical specialties. Unfortunately, ophthalmology is not one of the specific specialties. The AMA's contribution is significant because it examines the factors affecting the decision to attend medical school, rather than other postgraduate programs, and the choice of medical specialty. Current and past utilization trends are used to assess the level of demand for medical services; no estimates of the public health need for care are included in the model.

The foundation of the AMA workforce model is a statistical analysis of the supply and demand for services. For a select number of specialties (not including ophthalmology), the AMA regression models included factors believed to affect supply and demand, including aggregate economic factors and patient income. Thus, while the AMA model incorporates factors that are known to have an economic influence on supply and demand (a characteristic that sets it apart from other models), it assumes that utilization and demand patterns will follow historical trends. Consequently, there is limited flexibility to forecast workforce responses to major changes in historical trends.

Population-to-Workforce Ratio Studies

Recently, several studies have used the staffing ratios (physician-to-enrollee population) of health maintenance organizations (HMOs) to determine the level of medical workforce required in the United States. Such studies concluded that there is a large surplus of general specialists and surgical specialists, including ophthalmologists (Mulhausen and McGee, 1989; Kronick et al., 1993; Weiner, 1994). Staffing ratios implicitly reflect the use of nonphysician providers, which is particularly relevant to ophthalmology, in which ophthalmologists and optometrists can perform many of the same patient care tasks.

Using HMO workforce-to-population ratios, however, means that the requirements are based on demand within a certain health care delivery system; HMOs staff their plans to satisfy *current* utilization patterns. These ratios are one step removed from the direct utilization measurements used in the BHPr and AMA studies, or the theoretical requirements patterns used in the GMENAC study. In addition, studies using a workforce-to-population ratio approach cannot be directly generalized to the nation as a whole, because certain rural areas of the country have population densities that cannot support staff model HMOs (Kronick et al., 1993). Finally, age distributions and other population characteristics of HMO enrollees may limit the generalizability of using HMO staffing ratio models for the general population, although statistical adjustments can be made to improve estimates (Weiner, 1994).

ANALYSIS OF APPROACHES

Each of the models described above is a result of numerous decisions and assumptions about workforce supply and requirements. Choice and use of assumptions are critical in any workforce study (Feil et al., 1993; Rivo et al., 1993). One important consideration in calculating the requirements for services is whether current and past utilization patterns *(demand)* or population-based disease or condition incidence and prevalence rates *(need)* form the basis for the estimates. *From a public health perspective, meeting the need for care is the desired goal.* Utilization/demand is subject to patient demographic characteristics such as age, ethnicity, and health-specific knowledge, and to socioeconomic characteristics such as income and health insurance coverage that are subject to significant change, particularly under health care reform. Further, demand can reflect overutilization as well as underutilization. Attempts to estimate requirements according to "best practice standards" (i.e., current norms of care) are difficult when using utilization data. From another perspective, demand can be derived from need estimates adjusted for factors such as access, income, and insurance, *but true need cannot be readily calculated from demand.* Only the GMENAC study (and the derivative AAO study) proceeds from a needs-based approach and attempts to incorporate best practice standards through the use of specialty advisory panels. The BHPr and AMA models are demand-based studies.

Staffing ratio models are less precise than models based on utilization patterns or need. However, they may be more appropriate when there are insufficient data to estimate need or demand. When sufficient data exist, more detailed models that rely on a need- or demand-based approach can be used, with the dual advantage of explicitly incorporating those factors that determine workforce considerations and providing the flexibility to enable policymakers to project the possible effects of changes in specific factors.

The assumptions related to workforce supply and productivity--how personnel are trained and enter into practice, and the typical patient capacity that is offered--can similarly affect the results of the model. Most physician workforce studies make certain assumptions concerning the entry rates into the medical profession and into subspecialties; for example, the AAO study of the need for ophthalmologists assumed *entry* to be equivalent to the number of residency positions available and the number of FMGs entering ophthalmology to be minimal. Perhaps most significant, all models except the GMENAC share the shortcoming of not addressing the potential uses of nonphysician providers of care. Thus, the GMENAC approach is consistent with understanding the increasingly prominent role played by optometrists and other providers of eye care in addition to ophthalmologists.

Since the GMENAC study, numerous findings in the scientific literature have the potential to greatly improve contemporary workforce estimates. For example, several studies have reported population-based estimates of the incidence and prevalence of certain common eye diseases and conditions; diagnostic and therapeutic procedures have improved; and certain data collection systems enable a more detailed description and specification of the number of diseases that can be explicitly used in estimating the demand for eye care services. Such improvements add greater precision to the estimates and enable clearer distinctions to be made between the intensity of services that may be required from various eye care professionals. The presence of this greater specificity and precision lends itself to incorporation of both the GMENAC needs-based and BHPr minutes-based approaches to reconciling the available supply of eye care providers and requirements for care.

CURRENT ISSUES

Although the GMENAC study presents broad-based concepts of supply and requirements, major changes in the health care system have occurred since that study that affect both the supply and requirements for eye care and for eye care professionals. First, HMOs and other forms of managed care have, in general, become much more common. Such organizational forms can take advantage of the potential complementarity and possible substitutability of ophthalmologists, optometrists, and other professionals in specified areas. These types of care models have implications for the use of a variously composed workforce, and hence, implications for the workforce estimates.

Second, optometry has become much more prominent as a deliverer of eye care services. Since the 1980s, many changes have occurred in licensing and insurance benefits, expanding the role of optometrists in eye care and enlarging the numbers of eye care professionals available to provide specific types of care. Licensure changes highlight the need for flexibility in how provider time is allocated across condition/disease and supply categories in workforce estimates.

Third, productivity has changed. Certain surgical advances have made such procedures as cataract removal less time-consuming. In addition, workforce demographics are different. Shifts in age distribution, either to younger or older physicians, may cause the level of productivity to decrease: the youngest physicians are often in training and less productive, and the oldest physicians may be close to retirement and thus tapering off their work hours.

Fourth, population changes and changes in disease prevalence (e.g., AIDS) have occurred that affect workforce requirements. For ophthalmology, an aging population may be especially significant because older patients are the largest proportion of patients seen in ophthalmology practices and they have both a higher need and a higher demand for services.

Fifth, as with managed care, health care reform has the potential to affect medical practice in many ways. If health care reform affects the structure of medical care delivery through the use of primary care providers, such as in HMOs, in which generalist physicians may be used first, then referral patterns will change. To the extent other, substitute providers are available, the number of ophthalmologists required may decline. Also, to the extent that health care reform changes reimbursement rates, and hence income, the number of persons who go into ophthalmology and the number of hours worked per individual ophthalmologist also may change over time. Moreover, health care reform may alter the number of supported residency and fellowship positions: virtually all current reform proposals cite a perceived excess of subspecialty physicians and outline funding priorities for graduate medical education different from those used today.

Therefore, it is not surprising that a recent review of workforce studies over the last 20 years concluded that there is no generally accepted methodology for forecasting requirements for physicians over time, although the measurement of entrance and exit rates is a generally accepted approach for forecasting supply (Feil et al., 1993). Even in forecasting supply, significant variation can arise; in the 1970s, Reinhardt noted that as small a difference as 2 percent in the productivity growth of physicians would, over 10 years, lead to a 70,000-physician difference in estimates of the number of total physicians available (Reinhardt, 1973). Thus, although supply models are often the most developed, the robustness of workforce models depends on the comprehensiveness of the variables included in the modeling and the accuracy of the underlying assumptions and the projected values for each variable.

To reconcile these issues and those raised in the current health care policy debate, we examined the supply of eye care providers and the needs and demands for services under three different health care delivery scenarios. The first is what we call the *optometry-first* model, in which we assume that optometrists provide all primary eye care services and treat patients medically for their eye condition within current patterns of treatment. The second model, the ophthalmologist analog, we call the *ophthalmology-first* model, in which we assume that ophthalmologists provide all the primary eye care services, including medical and surgical treatment of a condition that they are capable of providing. The last we call the *primary care provider* model, in which optometrists and general ophthalmologists provide primary eye care services and general ophthalmologists provide the bulk of the medical and surgical treatment of eye conditions. Specialist ophthalmologists are used only for the surgical treatment of certain specialty-specific eye conditions. Estimates under these three delivery-system scenarios will fall within a range that reflects certain staffing and cost-containment concerns and that, consequently, will provide information to inform the current policy debate.

SUMMARY

This review of prior workforce studies discusses the range of possible approaches for estimating the supply and demand and need for eye care providers. Using data and methods not available to earlier studies, we can construct a needs-based model that is more detailed and accurate than the GMENAC. At the same time, the greater degree of precision resulting from improved data and methods enhances the attractiveness of the BHPr minutes-based approach. Finally, given the uncertainties of health care reform, *estimating both the need and demand for services addresses the range of issues currently being discussed in the health care policy debate.*

This report is structured to present first the methods and then the results of this workforce study. Chapter Two describes the conceptual framework of the study, outlines the models used for the supply, demand, and need for eye care providers, reviews the data and data sources used, and highlights issues that are addressed in succeeding chapters. Chapter Three describes the supply models for ophthalmologists and optometrists. Chapter Four addresses the requirements for eye care providers by quantifying the need for eye care services as well as the demand for such services. The reconciliation of provider supply with need and demand is elaborated in Chapter Five. Chapter Six summarizes our findings and discusses their policy implications.

2. THE MODEL: ISSUES AND CONCEPTUAL FRAMEWORK

INTRODUCTION

The models of eye care supply and requirements (need and demand) utilize eight steps to arrive at their output: counts of full-time equivalent (FTE) providers (optometrists, other physicians, and ophthalmologists, by specialty). Throughout this discussion, the use of the term FTE is meant to facilitate understanding of workforce interests and does not imply an equivalence in quality of care, cost, or cost-effectiveness. The eight steps are as follows:

1. Organize eye care services (diagnosis and procedure codes) into groupings, using a general domains-of-care framework.
2. Survey publicly available data for supply, demand, and need.
3. Establish population-based rates for requirements: utilization rates for demand, incidence and prevalence rates for need.
4. Conduct surveys to obtain data for clinical care requirements and work-time estimates.
5. Calculate available full-time equivalent (FTE) provider supply.
6. Calculate FTE providers required and reconcile with FTE supply.
7. Address data limitations and data uncertainties.
8. Project supply and need into the future.

Eye care encompasses a variety of diseases and conditions, and it is provided in many settings and by different types of providers. We developed a general conceptual framework to organize the breadth of eye care conditions and related services. Because development and implementation of the conceptual framework involved numerous decisions, we established an advisory panel to review our approach and data collection efforts. We also elicited and received input from various ophthalmology subspecialty societies. Our efforts were constrained by the nonparticipation of the American Optometric Association (AOA); the AOA was invited to participate in the study but declined.

This chapter describes the development of the conceptual framework used for this study. It then discusses each step of the model, focusing on specific decision points, analytic tasks, and general approaches to those tasks. The technical discussion of methods for computing supply, need, and demand are presented in Chapters Three and Four, respectively.

DOMAINS OF EYE CARE SERVICES

Workforce estimates have traditionally included only *problem-oriented* medical care--the diagnosis and treatment of physical maladies or problems--as practiced by physicians. Such estimates are broadened here to encompass three other aspects of care:

- Requirements for *preventive care*--periodic well-eye visits, or visits to detect early disease. The time needed to provide such care in accordance with recognized guidelines has generally not been explicitly incorporated into workforce estimates.

- Requirements for *rehabilitative* services. For those patients in which preventive and medical care have not been successful, helping patients adjust to a chronic condition and perhaps to lessen, if not reverse, its associated effects has significant value.

- Requirements for *elective* services. Workforce planning should at least be aware that many services provided by physicians and other health care providers may not fall into commonly accepted paradigms or conceptualizations as indicated by medical, preventive, or rehabilitative domains. In eye care, such services include the fitting of cosmetic contact lenses and refractive surgery. Elective services are considered by patients as having such sufficient value that many providers spend a significant portion of their time providing them.

Thus, we envision four domains of eye care services: problem-oriented, rehabilitative, preventive, and elective. This framework permits the constellation of eye care services to be partitioned into four domains that are, to a large extent, mutually exclusive. Patients who are being followed for problem-oriented or rehabilitative care should generally not also be counted as needing additional preventive care; we assume that their ongoing eye-care health needs are being met during their treatment visits. However, elective care patients may seek additional care, and they are not excluded from the other domains.

The present study uses the four-domain framework to better identify the contributions of the various types of providers and to provide insight into the workforce required to meet the needs and demands of each of these distinct domains. To begin identifying the differences, we turn to the first step of the model, a means of organizing the diseases, conditions, and diagnosis and procedure codes used in currently available sources of data on eye conditions and eye care services.

STEP 1. ORGANIZE DIAGNOSIS AND PROCEDURE CODES BY DOMAINS OF CARE

As with traditional workforce approaches, we focused initially on the medical, or problem-oriented, domain of care, because it is generally seen as the largest of the four domains and arguably the most important. Most national health care databases use diagnostic or procedure codes to describe a patient's condition. The thousands of diagnosis codes and procedure codes that can be used for eye care services necessitated organizing the codes into groups that were clinically distinct yet analytically manageable. We reviewed each of the potential eye diagnosis codes in the *International Classification of Diseases,* Ninth Revision (ICD-9), and assigned it to a disease group. This assignment was 1:1-that is, no ICD-9 diagnosis code was assigned to more than one disease group. During this process we separated those diagnostic codes describing diseases and conditions leading to rehabilitative care from those using problem-oriented services. This classification effort resulted in 93 disease groups for problem-oriented care and 4 disease groups for rehabilitative services. We further organized the 93 problem-oriented disease groups into 14 disease categories and the 4 rehabilitative disease groups into one specific category. This structure is illustrated in Figure 2.1, and the groups

and categories are listed in Table 2.1 (see Appendix A for a more
detailed discussion).

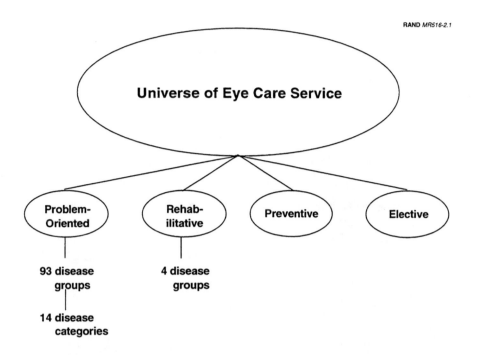

Fig. 2.1--Domains of Eye Care Services, With Disease Groups
and Categories

Table 2.1
Problem-Oriented and Rehabilitative Categories and Groupings of Care

1. Cataract
   a. cataract   c. aphakia/pseudophakia
   b. lens-related diseases   d. congenital cataract

2. Conjunctival disease
   a. severe conjunctivitis   c. conjunctival hemorrhage
   b. conjunctivitis

3. Cornea
   a. corneal infection   d. corneal dystrophy
   b. immune keratitis   e. corneal opacity
   c. corneal edema   f. corneal deposits

Note: Table continues on next page.

Table 2.1
Problem-Oriented and Rehabilitative Categories and Groupings of Care
(continued)

4. External disease and ocular
   surface
   a. blepharitis
   b. dry eye
   c. chalazion
   d. pterygium
   e. eyelid dermatitis
   f. trichiasis
   g. corneal/conjunctival mass

5. Glaucoma
   a. open-angle glaucoma
   b. glaucoma suspect
   c. narrow-angle glaucoma
   d. secondary glaucoma
   e. congenital glaucoma

6. Low vision[1]
   a. blindness
   b. color blindness
   c. one-eyed
   d. visual impairment

7. Neuro-Ophthalmology
   a. optic neuropathy
   b. visual disturbance
      (symptom)
   c. visual-field defect
   d. cranial nerve abnormality
   e. other central nervous system
   f. pupil abnormality
   g. optic nerve abnormality
   h. nystagmus

8. Orbital
   a. eyelid tumor
   b. orbital inflammation
   c. lacrimal gland disease
   d. orbital mass
   e. orbital deformity

9. Plastics
   a. external burns
   b. stenosis naso-lacrimal
      system
   c. ptosis
   d. dacrocystitis
   e. ectropion
   f. entropion
   g. external anomalies
   h. other tear duct abnormality
   i. conjunctival scarring
   j. other lid disease

10. Refractive
    a. myopia
    b. other refractive error
       (including presbyopia)
    c. astigmatism

Note: Table continues on next page.

Table 2.1
Problem-Oriented and Rehabilitative Categories and Groupings of Care
(continued)

11. Retinal
    a. macular degeneration
    b. diabetes
    c. retinal detachment
    d. vitreous opacities

    e. retinal degeneration

    f. arterial occlusion
    g. macular pucker
    h. central retinal vein
       occlusion/branch retinal
       vein occlusion
    i. chorioretinitis
    j. vitreous deposit
    k. retinal tumor

    l. choroidal tumor
    m. macular edema
    n. macular cyst/hole
    o. retinal vascular disease(non-
       occlusive)
    p. retinal pigment epithelial
       disorders (other)
    q. endophthalmitis
    r. retinopathy of prematurity
    s. intraocular anomalies

    t. exudative retinopathy
    u. HIV

12. Strabismus
    a. esotropia
    b. exotropia
    c. other and unspecified
       strabismus

    d. vertical strabismus
    e. amblyopia

13. Trauma
    a. superficial trauma
    b. superficial foreign body
    c. trauma--deep/foreign body
       (intraocular)
    d. trauma--deep/orbital

    e. sequelae trauma
    f. ruptured globe
    g. vitreous hemorrhage

    h. hypotony

14. Uveitis
    a. iridocyclitis
    b. posterior uveitis

    c. scleritis

15. Other
    a. herpes simplex
    b. herpes zoster
    c. iris lesions

    d. other ocular infections
    e. other

[1]Rehabilitative category. All others are problem-oriented.

These groupings reflect traditional diagnostic groupings, although with some variation from the ICD-9 coding system. Moreover, the aggregate categories tend to follow ophthalmological subspecialty lines, which facilitates extension of the workforce study to subspecialties.

Companion information to the classification of diagnosis codes is the classification of surgical procedure information, because the treatment of many eye diseases/conditions requires surgical intervention. Thus, it was necessary to assign procedure codes to disease groups. However, unlike diagnosis codes that relate only to one condition entity, procedures may be used to treat a variety of conditions. Thus, the assignment of procedure codes to condition entities was not 1:1; procedure codes can relate to two or more condition groups.

The process of assigning procedures to conditions was very detailed, but was facilitated by the disaggregation of the four domains. Ophthalmic procedure codes are from two different classification systems; these codes are either ICD-9 *(International Classification of Diseases, Ninth Revision)* or CPT-4 *(Physicians' Current Procedure Terminology, Fourth Edition)* codes or modifications of them. The ICD-9 is more physiologically based; the CPT-4 is more service based.

Finally, this clustering of diagnoses and procedures enabled us to distinguish medical and surgical treatment for a given episode of care. This distinction is important for two main reasons. First, the types of providers who can perform medical treatment for eye care conditions include ophthalmologists, optometrists, and other physicians, whereas only physicians (ophthalmologists and others, e.g., neurosurgeons) can perform the surgical procedures. Thus, our analysis of the supply of providers exploits this medical/surgical distinction. Second, the resources required differ between medical and surgical care. Generally, surgical care requires more time and more sophisticated equipment than medical treatment. The models thus include as separate surgical procedures only those procedures requiring significant additional resources of time and are not included as part of a usual office evaluation in the preceding clusters. Thus, for example, refraction, visual field examinations, or photography are not separately.included in the procedure groupings, while laser capsulotomy is.

STEP 2. SURVEY AVAILABLE DATA

Two decisions guided the models' structure and our attempts to gather data to support the models. First, because the models were to relate to clinical practice, we used the domains-of-care organization discussed in the prior section. Second, because the models were to be data-driven, we identified what data were readily available to support the models and where data collection efforts were required. Numerous data sources were used to develop the eye care workforce estimates; they correspond directly to the supply, demand, and need for services.

Supply

To determine current and future supply of FTE eye care providers, we obtained data from professional association membership databases and from Bureau of the Census surveys. The issue of the supply of eye care professionals not only involves the absolute number of professionals but also training characteristics, demographics, geographic distribution, and productivity information. The available data sources listed in Table 2.2 provided sufficient information on provider demographics and geographic location but not on productivity (e.g., the time it takes to care for a patient with a given disease, the number of disease-specific follow-up visits required, etc.). To obtain productivity information, we surveyed practicing ophthalmologists; the survey is described later in this chapter. The discussion that follows provides details about each data source.

Table 2.2
Data for Supply Estimation

Data Set
American Academy of Ophthalmology--Membership Master File
Ophthalmology Matching Program
AMA *Physician Characteristics and Distribution in the U.S.*
AMA *Physician Marketplace Statistics*
Area Resource File
Public Use Micro Sample (PUMS) Census Files

American Academy of Ophthalmology--Member Master File. The
American Academy of Ophthalmology provided its most recent (1993)
membership file, which consists of information reported by the members
that is updated periodically, as well as nonmember information, albeit a
limited-variable set, used for membership recruiting. This file
provides demographic information (age and gender), geographic location
(zip code and state), training information (year graduated, board
certification status), clinical preference (self-designated specialty),
and medical practice type (solo, health maintenance organization, etc.).
The AAO estimates that over 95 percent of all ophthalmologists are
represented in the data file because it includes both member and
nonmember ophthalmologists.

Ophthalmology Match Program. The Ophthalmology Match Program data
maintained by the Association of University Professors of Ophthalmology
provides information concerning the number of residency and fellowship
positions and applicants for the nation. These data indicate that
virtually all positions are filled, and numerous applicants remain
unmatched--a trend that has persisted over the past 15 years.

AMA Data. The American Medical Association annually surveys a
member sample to determine current practice characteristics. Some of
the information is reported by specialty, and some is reported by
geographic region. From *Physician Characteristics and Distribution in
the U.S.* (AMA, 1993b), we verified information concerning the age and
gender distribution of ophthalmologists for the nation, and the number
of ophthalmologists by major professional activity for the nation,
census region, and state. From the AMA's *Physician Marketplace*

Statistics (AMA, 1993c), we obtained information profiling
ophthalmologic practice: information concerning the average number of
weeks worked, hours per week spent in patient care, number of office
visits, number of surgeries, and other practice characteristics.

Area Resource File (AMA data). The Area Resource File (ARF, 1992)
is prepared by the Bureau of Health Professions and consists of data
from numerous secondary sources, including the American Medical
Association. This file has county-specific records detailing the number
of ophthalmologists by type of activity (patient care, hospital-based,
research, administration, etc.) and by age category (0-35, 35-44, 45-54,
55-64, 65+). We checked data from the 1992 ARF with state totals from
AMA-published materials; these numbers were the same. However, the ARF
counts were 11 percent less than the AAO counts and were systematically
under AAO counts within states; 47 of 50 states had lower ARF counts.
We believe that the AAO data are more complete, inasmuch as they form
the basis of communication between the AAO and practicing
ophthalmologists. Thus, we used the AAO data in developing our
ophthalmologist supply numbers.

Public Use Micro Sample (PUMS) Census Files. These data derive
from the 5 percent sample of households in the 1990 census that received
a detailed questionnaire, the so-called *long form*. These data, stripped
of identifying information, include occupational, demographic, and
geographic information, which enabled us to estimate the number of
optometrists by age, gender, and state.

Demand

The demand for services is reflected in the amount of care actually
obtained by patients--utilization. Three sources were reviewed against
our disease- and rehabilitation-based organization categories, and are
listed in Table 2.3. Other data sources, such as the National Medical
Expenditure Survey, were not included because they did not provide the
clinical information required for our model structure.

Table 2.3
Data for Demand Estimation

Data Set	Years
National Ambulatory Medical Care Survey	1989-1991
National Hospital Discharge Survey	1986, 1988-1990
National Health Interview Survey	1989, 1990

National Ambulatory Medical Care Survey. The National Ambulatory Medical Care Survey (NAMCS) is periodically conducted by the National Center for Health Statistics (NCHS). Samples of patient records are selected from a national sample of office-based physicians. Hospital clinics, community mental health centers, ambulatory surgery centers, and emergency rooms are not included in the sample, and nonphysician providers such as optometrists are not included. However, an analysis for the Bureau of Health Professions conducted by VHI indicated that overall less than 3 percent of overall physician visits are not captured in the NAMCS (Lewin, 1992). We reexamined these data and determined that less than 6 percent of eye visits occur in these other, non-physician office settings.

The NAMCS collects information concerning patient demographics and clinical condition, as well as physician specialty. Thus, the data from this survey provide a picture of the types of diseases treated by ophthalmologists, as well as the specialties of other physicians who treat eye conditions. NAMCS, while limited in treatment settings and provider types, permits demand for eye care services to be estimated by physician specialty. In addition, the NAMCS office-visit record indicates whether the visit is for a new condition or one that has been seen before the sampled visit. Thus, it was possible to develop estimates of "new" (i.e., incident) and "old" (i.e., prevalent) numbers of people by disease.

National Hospital Discharge Survey. The National Hospital Discharge Survey (NHDS) annually samples hospital discharges. The importance of this file to understanding the demand for eye care services has declined because the vast majority of ophthalmic surgery and care has moved to ambulatory settings. The survey, nonetheless, provides counts of discharges by patient characteristics by disease and procedure code and is useful for certain conditions (e.g., trauma).

National Health Interview Survey. The National Health Interview Survey (NHIS) is a household survey that asks respondents to self-report information concerning health status and health care utilization. This survey provided information by patient demographic characteristics by census region for eye disease or infirmity (prevalence) and visits by provider types (physicians by specialty, optometrists, etc.).

Need

The need for eye care service--the amount of care required to monitor or treat (ameliorate or cure) a condition or disease--is clear for problem-oriented and rehabilitative services, which by definition are disease- or condition-focused. For other types of care, such as preventive services, professional practice standards for preventive services may define need. For elective services, need is not defined; however, a patient may initiate "need" by electing to be fitted for contact lenses. Thus, we use demand as equivalent to need for elective services. Table 2.4 identifies the various sources of information available for estimates of need.

Table 2.4
Data for Need Estimation

Source
Census population projections

Common ophthalmic diseases
    Framingham Eye Study
    Baltimore Eye Study
    Beaver Dam Eye Study

Less common ophthalmic diseases
    Scientific literature
    [Demand-based adjustments using:
    National Health Interview Survey,
    National Hospital Discharge Survey,
    National Ambulatory Medical Care Survey]

Preventive and elective services
    AAO Preferred Practice Patterns
    National Eye Care Forum preventive care recommendations

Two types of information are required in order to assess the need for care. First, we require population-based epidemiological data concerning the incidence and prevalence of eye disease. In order to understand and identify the course of the disease, these data are often reported by age, gender, and race. Second, we require population information by the same demographic characteristics as those used by the epidemiological data. Moreover, the population estimates must be disaggregated by geographic units for regional estimates of need.

Census Population Projections. Whether epidemiologically based or guideline-based, our estimates of need require population counts or projections by the relevant demographic characteristics, such as age, race, and gender. The Bureau of the Census Projections file provided population estimates through the year 2010, by demographic characteristics and by state.

Common Ophthalmic Diseases Or Conditions. For problem-oriented services, we reviewed the literature for incidence and prevalence rates, by demographic characteristics, for eye conditions. The primary sources of this information are the Framingham, Baltimore, and Beaver Dam Eye Studies, whose rates vary according to the clinical definition used in

each study. To select the appropriate rates, we attempted to use the
definitions that were most consistent with our other data requirements
for the model or that were most consistent with current medical
practice. Where rates were available by demographic factors (e.g., race
and gender), we utilized the demographic factors available to create
more precise estimates. Judgment was often required in deciding how to
impute prevalence and incidence rates for ages outside the ranges
established by the large eye studies. For younger ages, if the rate was
known to be zero for some specified age, we smoothly interpolated from
that age to the earliest age for which rates were available. For older
ages, we generally set the rate equal to the value for the oldest age
available. To ensure that our estimates of need were at least
commensurate with estimates of demand, we compared our estimates with
the utilization estimates of national prevalence and incidence derived
from NAMCS (three survey years, 1989-1991, were combined).

Less Common Ophthalmic Diseases. For less common ophthalmic
diseases, such as pupil abnormality, we used disease-specific estimates
from smaller studies reported in the scientific literature. If no data
were available, we used our estimates of demand as the starting point
for estimates of need. We then scaled those estimates to reflect need,
because demand, as measured from national utilization surveys,
represents only that fraction of people with disease who seek treatment.
We did this scaling by finding a similar disease or disease grouping for
which the need-to-demand ratio could be computed (i.e., data available
for both need and demand) and scaled by that ratio for the condition in
question (see the next section).

Preventive and Elective Services. For preventive services, we
relied on the AAO Preferred Practice Pattern for well-eye exams for
adults. For children and infants, we used the AAO-sponsored March 1994
National Eye Care Forum Consensus Conference recommendations (Table
2.5). The Forum reached a consensus view of reasonable schedules for
eye care examinations; the view represented industry, managed care,
government, and consumer interests. However, the AOA has subsequently
withdrawn its support of the Forum's recommendations, in part because it
believes that the frequency of visits in the Forum Consensus Conference

recommendations is too low for all ages. Our estimates of preventive services thus use the more liberal AAO Preferred Practice Patterns as opposed to the National Eye Care Forum recommendations for adults. However, because no such practice patterns are available for infants and children, we elected to use the Forum recommendations for persons age 18 and under.

Table 2.5
National Eye Care Forum Preventive Eye Care Services Schedule

Summary of Group Consensus for
Individuals Without Signs or Symptoms of Disease

Age Group	Type of Service	Frequency
Perinatal	Screening	Once during period (birth-one month)
Infants	Screening	Once during period (1-11 months)
Early childhood	Exam	Once during period (1-5 years)
Childhood	Exam	Once every 2 years (6-10 years)
School Age	Screening	Twice during period (11-18 years)

Source: National Eye Care Forum Preventive Eye Care Services Schedule (AAO, 1994).

Because elective services are not generally covered by insurance, little information is available on utilization of such services. Much of the available data on eye care services are based on the ICD and CPT systems developed to help track services for reimbursement purposes. After discussion with numerous ophthalmologists and our advisory panel, we decided to define elective services narrowly and to include only those services for which some information is available. Thus, *elective services* include contact lens fitting and refractive surgery. For elective services, we used demand for care, as determined through surveys of utilization, subspecialty societies, and eye care product manufacturers' estimates. However, only a portion of the total services requirements for contact lens fitting is included in the elective services, because we assume that the majority of contact lens care is delivered in the course of routine care for "refractive error" (a condition category).

STEP 3. ESTABLISH POPULATION PREVALENCE, INCIDENCE, AND CLINICAL RATES

The third step was to identify sources of data that would provide information on the prevalence and incidence for our 97 groupings, along with an estimate of the population of persons with those diseases who would require care beyond that provided during routine well-eye exams according to the AAO Preferred Practice Patterns visit schedule. This task focussed mainly on deriving estimates for public health need. Demand rates were extrapolated directly from utilization.

Need--Prevalence and Incidence Rates

To obtain data on the need for eye care, we first obtained current and future population estimates from the U.S. Bureau of the Census. Then we obtained incidence and prevalence rates for eye diseases from the scientific literature. Three major ophthalmic epidemiological studies are described in the scientific literature: the Beaver Dam, Framingham, and Baltimore Eye Studies. These studies were population-based and provided detailed incidence and prevalence information for common ophthalmic diseases.[1]

Use of these studies presented three problems, however. First, although each of the studies was population-based, the populations studied were not nationally representative. For example, none of the studies has a significant Asian-American representation, and only the Baltimore Eye Study has a significant African-American representation. Second, the number of diseases for which incidence and prevalence information was obtained is fairly low. Third, while there is some overlap among the studies, their definitions of disease differ. For

---

[1]We decided not to use incidence and prevalence rates derived from the National Health and Nutrition Examination Survey (NHANES). These rates differed significantly from the rates obtained from the three major ophthalmic epidemiological studies. In addition, major organizations, such as Prevent Blindness America and The National Eye Institute, have decided to use the rates from the three ophthalmic epidemiological studies as the basis for their estimates.

example, the degree of opacity and visual or functional limitations (if any) required before a diagnosis of "cataract" is made varies across the three studies.

Thus, obtaining prevalence and incidence numbers for all 97 disease groupings required input from our advisory board of physicians. In addition, Prevent Blindness America furnished us their estimates of incidence or prevalence for five major eye conditions: cataract, glaucoma, macular degeneration, diabetic retinopathy, and visual impairment.

We used the following strategies to produce the incidence and prevalence rates for our models.

1. In all cases, we used the definitions that were most consistent with other data required for the model or that were most consistent with current medical practice.

2. While the scientific literature provided information on common eye conditions, it did not provide information for those diseases that are less common. Thus, for those conditions where population-based or other scientific study data were not available, we used estimates from the NAMCS as the starting point. We then rescaled those rates to need using a need-to-demand ratio from a disease group that was similar and also within the same disease category.

3. In using the NAMCS numbers, we attempted to estimate incidence and prevalence separately. Visits for a new condition were flagged, leading to simple estimates of incidence. For prevalence, we converted visits into numbers of people with the disease by using a data element recorded from our surveys of ophthalmologists (described below): the median number of disease-specific follow-up visits required per year. Dividing the number of visits by the number of median follow-up visits from our survey provided an estimate of the number of individuals with the particular disease or condition.

4. For those conditions that generally require hospitalization (e.g., significant trauma), we used the treatment numbers from

the National Hospital Discharge Survey as representative of
disease incidence. Because such conditions (or situations) are
acute, a zero prevalence rate was used. Sequelae related to
trauma are included in other disease codes. No scaling was
done since we assumed patients with these conditions would be
seen (i.e., demand equals need).

Table 2.6 displays the 15 disease and rehabilitative categories and
the types of information used in developing prevalence and incidence
information for each group. Figure 2.2 diagrams our model for
estimating need.

Need--Determination of Clinical Rates

Once we had established proper disease-specific incidence and
prevalence rates, we needed to determine what proportion of persons with
a given disease actually require care beyond the preventive care visit
schedules. We recognized that all persons with ophthalmic pathology
require some level of monitoring, but that only a certain proportion of
them would require more intense monitoring and treatment than would be
available during routine well-eye exams at specified intervals. As
such, it is only when a condition merits more careful or more frequent
monitoring or treatment, at specified levels generated from our survey
discussed in the following section and detailed in Chapter Four, that a
patient is included in the clinical population for one of the 97
groupings. Both the definition and the estimates of the disease-
specific clinical population were reviewed by our advisory panel of
ophthalmologists.

Table 2.6
Source of Incidence and Prevalence (Need) Information by Disease Category

Disease Category	Sources
01 Cataract	Beaver Dam Eye Study, Framingham Eye Study, Baltimore Eye Study, Prevent Blindness America, Duke-Elder
02 Conjunctivitis	NAMCS
03 Cornea	NAMCS (adjusted)
04 External disease	NAMCS (adjusted)
05 Glaucoma	Baltimore Eye Study, Framingham Eye Study, Prevent Blindness America
06 Rehabilitation	Baltimore Eye Study, Prevent Blindness America, Scientific literature
07 Neuro-ophthalmology	Scientific literature, NHIS, NAMCS (adjusted)
08 Orbital	NAMCS (adjusted)
09 Plastics	Scientific literature, NAMCS (adjusted)
10 Refractive	NHIS, Framingham Eye Study
11 Retina	Beaver Dam Eye Study, Framingham Eye Study, Prevent Blindness America, NHIS, Scientific literature, NAMCS (adjusted)
12 Strabismus	NHIS, Scientific literature, NAMCS (adjusted)
13 Trauma	NHIS, Scientific literature, NHDS, NAMCS (adjusted)
14 Uveitis	NAMCS (adjusted)
15 Other	NAMCS (adjusted)

RAND *MR516-2.2*

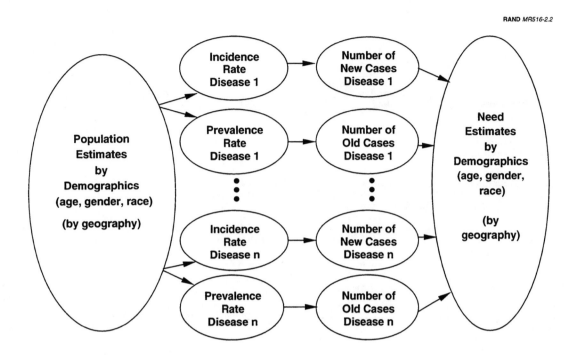

Fig. 2.2--Estimation of Population Need for Eye Care Services

Demand--Old and New Visit Rates

We modeled demand rates primarily from NAMCS and NHDS. NAMCS provided ambulatory medical visit rates for most conditions, as well as indicating whether the visit was for a new or old condition. The sampling design of NAMCS precluded significant information on trauma cases, which often require hospitalization. For those conditions involving hospitalization, we used NHDS to model demand. Figure 2.3 diagrams our model for estimating demand for eye care services. Again, our examination and reanalysis of the data presented in the VHI report suggests that less than 6 percent of the current utilization of eye care is missed by the NAMCS database due to survey design exclusions of non-office-based practice settings.

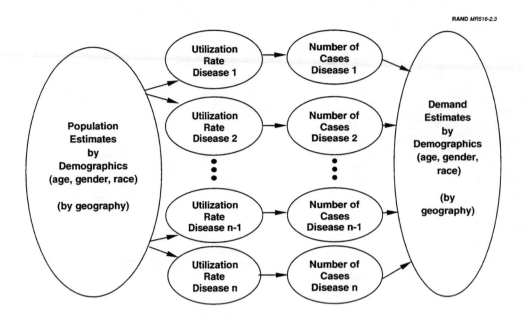

RAND MR516-2.3

Fig. 2.3--Estimation of Population Demand for Eye Care Services

Preventive and Elective Rates

Preventive and elective services are clearly important forms of care. Generally, they are not captured in most utilization surveys. We chose to adopt a standard for preventive care--the AAO Preferred Practice Patterns visit schedule for adults and the National Eye Care Forum recommendations for children--which enabled us to estimate FTE requirements for preventive care. Elective surgery (i.e., refractive surgery and contact lens problem rates) were estimated on the basis of summary figures presented by subspecialty societies, the AAO, and the AOA.

STEP 4. CONDUCT SURVEY OF WORKTIMES AND CLINICAL CARE REQUIREMENTS

Companion information to the number of patients requiring care is the estimated amount of time to treat the specific ophthalmic condition. Use of our model requires detailed estimates for each step of monitoring or treatment of a disease. Unfortunately, there is little disease-specific information that describes the amount of time for an initial visit and the number and length of follow-up medical visits, the proportion of patients who require surgical treatment, pre-operative assessment time, intra-operative time, other same-day surgical time, and the number and length of post-operative (i.e., 90-day) visits. Such information is required for a condition-based model of workforce requirements.

Some work-time information was available from the Health Care Finance Administration's resource-based relative value system for a small number of ophthalmic services and procedures (Hsiao et al., 1991). However, we did not use this information because of the small sample sizes used to determine the time estimates, the few procedures and services covered, and the lack of detailed information on office or medical care by condition.

The AAO produced work-time estimates in 1978 (Reinecke, 1978), as did GMENAC in 1981, for medical and surgical care for many of the disease groupings used in our study. We reviewed those estimates and found that the 1978 times were generally longer than what might be expected today, especially the surgical times. Similarly, the length of the average office visit also appeared to be longer than current practice. Because significant changes have occurred in ophthalmic practice in the intervening generation, we did not utilize information from these sources.

To compensate for the lack of current worktime information, we conducted a survey of ophthalmologists. To ensure that the survey met the disease-specific data needs of the study, we developed 10 ophthalmic subspecialty-specific surveys: cataract, cornea, glaucoma, low vision, neuro-ophthalmology, pediatrics and strabismus, oculo-plastics, retina, uveitis, and general ophthalmology. The combined disease and procedure lists from all surveys covered all of the 15 disease and rehabilitative categories, with an average of four disease groups within each category. The specific groupings surveyed included more than 95 percent of current utilization. There is partial overlap for certain common conditions and procedures, such as cataract and glaucoma. This survey, sent to a subspecialty-stratified random sample of 2,007 ophthalmologists, requested disease-specific time estimates as described above. From the 2,007 surveys, we obtained a 40 percent response rate. A full description of the development and implementation of the survey can be found in the companion report entitled *RAND Eye Care Workforce Survey* (forthcoming); the survey is discussed further in Chapter Four. Figure 2.4 is a sample of a page from the survey for general ophthalmologists.

Our survey obtained disease- and procedure-specific worktimes for each of the 97 eye conditions. The information obtained was stable across time (i.e., there was no response time bias), and our response rate was adequate to generate statistically stable work-time estimates (see Chapter Four for a more detailed discussion). Certain issues, such as the amount of time required for the administrative activities of care or continuing medical education, were explicitly not included in the survey. Although such activities directly affect the character of medical practice, the time devoted to such activities may differ by health care system or practice structure, systems that may change with health care reform. In contrast, the elements of care that were surveyed are common to *any* health care delivery system and are thus stable across delivery or financing systems.

STEP 5. CALCULATE AVAILABLE FTE PROVIDERS

We determined the number of eye care providers from professional association databases and from publicly available information, such as the census.

The subspecialty designation of ophthalmologists is made from self-reported information maintained by the AAO. Thus, we were able to determine the number of eye care providers (ophthalmologists and optometrists) by subspecialty (ophthalmologists) in such a way as to fit into our domains of care and disease groupings/categories (which relate directly to the types of services provided and ophthalmic subspecialty groups).

Other non-ophthalmologist physicians also provide eye care services. While we could determine their supply by using AMA information, we assumed that there will always be a sufficient supply of other physicians to provide the level of eye care services that they currently provide. Additional specification seemed inappropriate given that the services they provide for other, nonophthalmic diseases are not considered in this study.

SECTION 3: MEDICAL VISITS

Please complete the following table providing information concerning your **typical** patient. We are interested in obtaining data which reflect your experience in your practice. That is, provide the information only for those diagnoses you see in your practice and for which you feel comfortable providing estimates.

INITIAL VISITS

For example, in your practice you saw 10 new cataract patients in the last 30 days. The initial evaluation takes on average 35 minutes which is comprised of 20 minutes of your time, 5 minutes of technician's time, and 10 minutes of optometrist's time.

DIAGNOSIS	Your Practice (A) Estimate of **Number** of **NEW** patients seen in the last 30 days	Ophthalmologist Average length of **INITIAL** visit in minutes	Optometrist Average length of **INITIAL** visit in minutes	Registered Nurse Average length of **INITIAL** visit in minutes	Technician/ Technologist Average length of **INITIAL** visit in minutes
Cataract	10	20	10	0	5
CATARACT					
CONJUNCTIVITIS					
SEVERE CONJUNCTIVITIS					
OPEN-ANGLE GLAUCOMA					
REFRACTIVE ERROR / MYOPIA					
APHAKIA / PSEUDOPHAKIA					
MACULAR DEGENERATION					

Fig. 2.4--RAND Survey of Ophthalmologist Practice Patterns (sample page)

We estimated the number of training slots available, and we assumed
that each trainee provided a fraction of an FTE's worth of services. We
then converted the number of total FTEs into minutes of supply
availability using the 1993 AMA figure of 2,016 hours of direct patient
care per year, reported by ophthalmologists. As such, the approach
parallels the BHPr minutes-based method. See Figure 2.5 for a diagram
of our provider supply model.

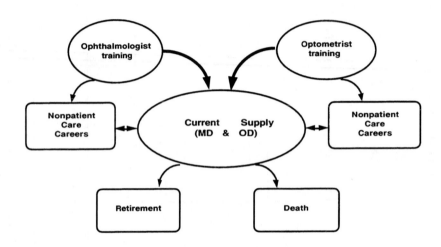

Fig. 2.5--Provider Supply Model

STEP 6. CALCULATE FTE REQUIREMENTS AND RECONCILE WITH FTE SUPPLY

The total number of FTE providers required to meet the need and
demand of the U.S. population is determined by the following equation:

Number of FTE providers$_i$ required =

{[Number of prevalence cases]$_i$ * [time to treat prevalence case]$_i$ +
　[Number of incidence cases]$_i$ * [time to treat incidence case]$_i$}

　　　　　　　　　[FTE conversion factor]

where i is one of the 97 groupings (and preventive and elective care),
prevalence and incidence cases are either database-centered estimates of

demand or the product of population sizes and the corresponding rates, [times to treat] are based on the ophthalmologist workforce surveys and used for both ophthalmologists and optometrists, and [FTE conversion factor] is the number of hours per year per provider, or 2,016 hours of patient care work per year.

The determination of which type of eye care provider used is a function not only of availability and patient preference but also regulation. Ophthalmologists can treat, either medically or surgically, any eye disease; optometrists are limited to medical treatment within certain prescribed boundaries (except for laser surgery, which is allowed in one state). The reconciliation of supply with need and of supply with demand is accomplished through a linear programming model that allocates providers to cases to maximize the level of provider training within groupings.

For this analysis, provider training is defined very narrowly. The lowest level is scored at 0, indicating that the provider type cannot legally treat a patient with this condition or provide surgical treatment. This score is used for optometrists who, in a limited number of situations, are prohibited by law from prescribing certain medication (e.g., systemic medication) or performing certain procedures (generally, surgical procedures). However, in identifying levels for which optometrists cannot provide treatment, we applied a standard consistent with the broadest optometric practice laws. We used this approach because it provides for the possibility of optometrists' obtaining expanded therapeutic privileges nationally.

All other provider scores are positive and are chosen so that the resulting allocations reveal the minimum and maximum possible uses of each type of provider. We varied these "training" scores to model different staffing preferences under three different health care delivery scenarios: optometrists allocated first to primary eye-care services; ophthalmologists allocated first to primary eye-care services; and a primary care provider model that uses optometrists and general ophthalmologists for providing primary eye-care services.

We wish to emphasize that we are not making estimates of quality of care or of cost-effectiveness but are only using legal privileges and training to guide the allocation of providers under different organizational schemes of care.

STEP 7. ADDRESS DATA LIMITATIONS AND DATA VARIATIONS
Limitations of the Data

The development of the workforce model for eye care professionals highlighted the paucity of data surrounding many of the variables we needed to include. Some of these data needs were satisfied through activities carried out by the project; other data needs were too extensive for this project to undertake and will remain for future research activities.

Population-based estimates of the incidence and prevalence of eye diseases were a major data deficiency of this project. Although scientifically based data permitted us to establish over 85 percent of the estimated public health need, the nonrepresentativeness of the populations sampled and the variation in the clinical definitions of disease used among the studies limits the precision of the model.

Second, there are limitations as to what we know about optometry's contribution to the provision of eye care services. We model optometry's provision of medical eye care to allow privileges consistent with the most broad-based state regulations. However, there are still many open questions as to how optometrists practice, how much time they take to provide these medical services, and how much time services not covered in this study consume in an optometrist's work year.

Third, an integral step in our public health need model is to define the number of persons with an eye condition who require, or *need*, care. The definition of the clinical population used in the study presented a problem because there are no data, that we are aware of, that translate incidence and prevalence into need for care. Unlike certain acute or infectious conditions (e.g., myocardial infarction or tuberculosis), many eye conditions do not medically require care.[2] We

---

[2]For example, although patients with subconjunctival hemorrhages rarely need to be seen by a physician, many patients seek reassurance from their physician. Consequently, the model does not have every patient with a subconjunctival hemorrhage being seen, but only a proportion of them.

implemented our definition of clinical population as a disease-specific fractional multiplier and applied it to the number of persons in the population with a particular condition (using incidence and prevalence information), thus yielding the number of persons needing disease-specific care, at levels determined through our survey.[3] Future studies need to address the issue of determining the number of persons with eye pathology that requires care at levels greater than those provided during a routine preventive eye care visit.

Fourth, estimates of the number of hours per FTE per year are subject to ongoing changes in our health care system. For our analyses, we used 2,016 hours of direct patient care per year (48 weeks of work times 42 hours per week). This number was selected after examining our survey results, comparing the survey result to similar data provided by the American Medical Association survey of medical practice, and discussing it (and its implications) with our advisory board. While 2,016 represented an estimate that the majority felt approximated reality, given the diversity of ophthalmic practice, there were arguments for both increasing and decreasing the number.

Methods for Addressing Data Limitations

In view of these four concerns, the myriad of variables contained in the models, and the use of data from disparate sources (i.e., different samples and surveys), we were concerned about the effect of data variability on the statistical stability of the results. To address these concerns, we used the "bootstrap," a statistical technique that resamples the data so that the model's calculations can be repeated and the results compared. In addition, we purposely introduced statistical perturbations (i.e., random statistical variation) in the

---

[3]The NHANES data set includes information that addresses the concept of clinical population in that it identifies patients, by disease, who need care. However, when these need rates were applied to our estimates of incidence and prevalence, the estimated need was far below estimates of current demand. Further, the clinical definitions used in the study differed from those used in current practice, and there are treatment approaches used today that were not available when the NHANES study was conducted. Ultimately, our advisory panel reviewed the clinical multipliers used in our models.

data to assess the robustness, or stability, of our results.. We were therefore able to generate a range of estimates that, as is shown in Chapter Five, indicate that the models' basic results are stable. Finally, we address some of the critical assumptions of the models and explore the effect of alternative assumptions on the results in Chapter Six. In this way, we can construct a measure of confidence in the study findings so that if questions are raised about the data in one particular cell or group of cells, we are confident that there is a small likelihood that adjustments to these data will significantly affect the overall results.

STEP 8. FUTURE PROJECTION

The final step in our analysis of the eye care services workforce was to make projections so that the excess or deficit of providers in the future could be assessed. The projections included assumptions about a population that will have a higher proportion of people over 65 than today's population (many eye care services are provided for age-related conditions; so as the U.S. population ages, the workforce picture will change as well). We also assumed that the supply of providers changes slowly because of the long time required for training and the many years individual providers are employed in the workforce. Thus, projections about the future embrace workforce concerns in addition to that of an assessment of current supply and requirements.

SUMMARY

This workforce study is framed by four domains of care: problem-oriented, rehabilitative, elective, and preventive services. These domains are defined by aggregates of clinical conditions to which diagnostic and procedure codes are assigned that parallel ophthalmology subspecialties and that permit the identification of medical and surgical components of care that parallel provider-specific treatment regimes. Structuring of the framework into diagnosis groupings subordinate to the domains of care enabled us to estimate the number of persons in need of treatment and the number of persons who currently receive treatment. The ophthalmologist survey, conducted specifically for this study, yields work-time estimates of FTE providers. These work-time estimates are applied to the number of persons needing care to obtain the number of providers needed. Reconciling the number of providers needed with the supply of providers generates estimates of an over- or undersupply of providers. These estimates can then inform the workforce policy debate. The next chapters provide detailed technical discussions of the methods used.

3. SUPPLY OF EYE CARE PROVIDERS

The many different types of health care providers perform similar (*substitutable*) or different (*complementary*) services in providing the range of available services defined in the four domains of care: elective, preventive, rehabilitative, and problem-oriented. Providers further vary in the length of time they work, the efficiency (time and quality) with which they take care of similar problems, the range of services which they provide, and their ability to deliver care independently without the assistance of other providers. Thus, measuring the available supply of providers of eye care goes beyond merely measuring the number of available individuals who are legally empowered to provide care.

In this study, we sought to identify in detail the supply of the providers who can independently provide some forms of eye care: ophthalmologists, optometrists, and other physicians. This chapter is organized in three sections, corresponding to these types of provider. We did not consider the supply of technicians, nurses, or assistants who support these independent providers of care nor did we consider the supply of receptionists or secretaries, because they can be considered to be drawn from the overall labor pool without significant barriers to entry influencing the available supply.

SUPPLY OF OPHTHALMOLOGISTS
Number of Ophthalmologists

To describe the supply of ophthalmologists, we utilized the American Academy of Ophthalmology (AAO) membership database as the primary source and the American Medical Association (AMA) Master File of Physicians and enumerations from the Area Resource File compiled by the Bureau of Health Professions as alternative sources. We selected the AAO database because we considered it the most complete and up-to-date file available. Comparison of the three data sources revealed that the number of ophthalmologists was greatest in the AAO database, suggesting a potential relative undercount in the other sources. Furthermore, more detailed data were available in the AAO database on the age, self-identified subspecialty or primary area of practice, fellowship subspecialty training, geographic location, and other practice details of the individual ophthalmologist, details that permitted more refined and detailed analyses.[4]

To calculate the number of available ophthalmologists in the United States, we obtained the number of active ophthalmologists by self-identified subspecialty practice, if any, from the AAO database. These numbers were tabulated by age, subspecialty, and geographic location for our projections. Table 3.1 displays the number of active ophthalmologists by area of subspecialization; however, these totals do not represent FTEs (see following sections).

Table 3.1
Number of Active Ophthalmologists (members and fellows),
by Subspecialty: 1994

Subspecialty	Number	Subspecialty	Number
General	8,399	Pediatrics	449
Cataract	2,282	Plastics	349
Cornea	915	Retina	1,169
Glaucoma	495	Uveitis	16
Low vision	8	Other	17
Neuro-Ophthalmology	126		
		Total	14,225

Source: AAO Membership Master File, 1994.

NOTE: Counts are for active ophthalmologists with known addresses, living in the United States.

Residents and Fellows in Training

Because our unit of workforce measure is a full-time equivalent (FTE) provider, we considered residents and fellows in ophthalmology as fractions of an FTE. The AMA annual survey of Graduate Medical Education Programs indicates there were 1,584 ophthalmology residents in

---

[4]Self-designation reflects training and what the physicians want to do, not necessarily what their practice consists of. Therefore, many subspecialists provide substantial amounts of general or comprehensive ophthalmology care.

135 ophthalmology residency programs in 1992. The Association of University Professors of Ophthalmology reports 496 residency positions available annually, with 487 filled, and 272 fellowship positions available annually, with 211 filled. We assumed that the entering cohort size each year is 487 and the length of residency training is three years (the number of four year programs is small). After the third year, we assumed that residents chose either to become general ophthalmologists or to develop additional skills in a subspecialty and pursue fellowship training. For purposes of computing current FTE ophthalmologists, we assumed that residents performed 35, 35, and 50 percent of an FTE's workload during years one, two, and three respectively.[5]

For fellows, we assumed that 250 fellowship slots (a compromise between the 272 available and 211 filed) are taken each year from the pool of residents who completed their third year. We distributed these slots among subspecialties in proportion to the current distribution of fellowship training slots, as shown in Table 3.2. We assumed that fellows performed 50 and 75 percent of an FTE subspecialist's workload during years one and two of their fellowship training. After two years of fellowship training, we assumed that fellows become full-fledged subspecialists.

Table 3.2
Distribution of Fellows, by Subspecialty: 1994

Specialty	Percentage	Specialty	Percentage
Cataract/external disease	12.4	Pediatrics	14.5
Cornea	25.0	Plastics	0.8
Glaucoma	16.6	Retina	27.9
Low vision	0.8	Uveitis	0.8
Neuro-Ophthalmology	1.2		

Source: Association of University Professors of Ophthalmology, *Match Report*, 1993.

---

[5]GMENAC used 35 percent for all years of residency and fellowship training.

Adjustments to the Number of Ophthalmologists

The number of ophthalmologists in full-time academic employment is 814. Because academic employment requires that time be spent in research and teaching, we included these ophthalmologists as 0.50 FTE and counted them in their particular subspecialty areas, when the information was available.[6] When subspecialty information was not available, we distributed the academic ophthalmologists proportionally across the subspecialty pool of active ophthalmologists (not including general ophthalmologists), since the vast majority of full-time academic ophthalmologists are subspecialists.

The RAND Eye Care Workforce Survey (RWS) revealed that about 4 percent of the ophthalmologists who were initially classified as "active" were in fact retired or deceased. We estimated these percentages within subspecialty and reduced the ophthalmologist population sizes accordingly.

The RWS also indicated that female ophthalmologists worked fewer hours than males: a median of 45 work hours per week for females, versus 50 for males. This finding is consistent with data reported from other workforce studies. The most recent AMA study on differences between female and male physicians (Schwartz et al., 1988) found that, overall, female physicians work 7.9 percent fewer hours per week, and have 18.5 percent fewer visits per week. Of surgical specialties, female physicians work .7 percent more hours per week but have 17.8 percent fewer visits. We wanted an adjustment that was consistent with these diverse findings, and assumed that female ophthalmologists provide 85 percent of an FTE. Use of a higher percentage would increase the supply of FTEs available.

Additional computations of ophthalmologists working part-time or sharing a position were not included because of the lack of data about such situations. Future workforce efforts may need to more explicitly consider these situations, and the AAO may wish to include questions about such arrangements in its annual membership data-collection

---

[6]GMENAC made no adjustment for academic physicians.

efforts. Otherwise, the number of ophthalmologists satisfying the FTE requirements may be overestimated.

Projecting the Supply of Ophthalmologists

We projected the number of FTE ophthalmologists during the years 1994 through 2010 in a series of six steps (see Table 3.3):

Table 3.3
Projected Number of Ophthalmologists: 1994-2010

| | Beginning-of-Year Status | | | End-of-Year Status | | |
Year	Full	In-Training	FTE Ophthal.	Full	In-Training Graduates	Total Ophthal.
1994	14,225	1,961	14,091	13,882	485	14,367
1995	14,367	1,958	14,215	13,907	484	14,391
1996	14,390	1,957	14,225	14,070	482	14,552
1997	14,553	1,957	14,370	14,238	482	14,720
1998	14,721	1,957	14,523	14,412	482	14,894
1999	14,894	1,957	14,677	14,580	482	15,062
2000	15,063	1,957	14,828	14,749	482	15,231
2001	15,232	1,957	14,979	14,917	482	15,399
2002	15,400	1,957	15,128	15,076	482	15,558
2003	15,558	1,957	15,270	15,230	482	15,712
2004	15,712	1,957	15,407	15,373	482	15,855
2005	15,855	1,957	15,533	15,503	482	15,985
2006	15,985	1,957	15,647	15,619	482	16,101
2007	16,102	1,957	15,748	15,723	482	16,205
2008	16,206	1,957	15,838	15,813	482	16,295
2009	16,295	1,957	15,913	15,888	482	16,370
2010	16,370	1,957	15,974	15,950	482	16,432

1. At the beginning of a year, we counted the number of ophthalmologists, residents, and fellows, by subspecialty. We allocated a fraction of residents and fellows to the FTE workforce supply, depending on where they are in their training cycle.

2. During a year, ophthalmologists, residents, and fellows retire or die at age- and gender-specific rates, which are drawn from the BHPr (Greenberg, 1992).

3. After their third year, residents graduate and become either
    full-FTE general ophthalmologists or fellows in subspecialty
    areas.

4. After their fellowship years, fellows graduate and become full-
    FTE ophthalmologists in their subspecialty areas.

5. A cohort of new residents in ophthalmology is registered into
    its first year.

6. We iterated these steps out to the year 2010.

Work-Time Estimates

Information on the annual medical practice time of ophthalmologists
was obtained from the RAND Eye Care Workforce Survey (RWS). The RWS is
a probability sample, stratified by subspecialty type, of active
ophthalmologists. Most of the survey focused on obtaining data needed
to calculate the requirements for eye care providers (detailed in
Chapter Four).

Because our survey results of the hours worked each year
potentially include administrative time and time spent in care not
directly related to direct patient care time (such as obtaining pre-
authorization), we also evaluated the results of the AMA annual survey
of physician work time (looking only at ophthalmologists), which has
detailed data on how time is spent. As seen in Table 3.4, the AMA
survey's median number of work weeks per year is similar to that of the
RAND survey (48) and the aggregate number of hours in patient care is
also very similar (AMA 46 versus RWS 50). However, including only the
number of patient visit hours and time in the operating room (42) in the
AMA study results in a direct patient care time that is 84 percent of
RWS. The 16 percent difference was identified by consulting
ophthalmologists and the advisory panel as being a realistic reflection
of physician time spent in nondirect patient care. However, this may
vary by system of care (e.g., prior authorization).

Table 3.4
AMA Work Time Data: FTE Definition

Activity	Median
Weeks of Practice, 1992	48.0
Hours in All Professional Activities per Week, 1993	52.0
Hours in Patient Care Activities per Week, 1993	46.0
Total Patient Visit Hours per Week, 1993	36.0
Office Hours per Week, 1993	35.0
Hours on Hospital Rounds per Week, 1993	0.0
Hours in Outpatient Clinics and Emergency Rooms per Week, 1993	0.0
Hours in Surgery per Week, 1993	6.0
RAND Eye Care Workforce Survey: Weeks of Practice	48.0
RAND Eye Care Workforce Survey: Work Hours per Week	50.0

Source: American Medical Association, *Physician Marketplace Statistics*, 1993.

For our analyses, we used 48 weeks of work, and 42 hours per week (total patient visit hours per week plus hours in surgery per week) as the amount of patient contact time, which yields 2,016 hours of direct patient care per year. This figure is close to that used by the GMENAC study--1950.5 annual hours worked (47 weeks, 41.5 hours per week). The prior AAO (1978-1984) study estimated 1,794 annual hours worked (46 weeks, 39 hours per week), based on a survey of members (Worthen et al., 1981). Thus, we and the advisory panel believe the figure used in our study represents a realistic estimate of the currently available patient care work time for an FTE ophthalmologist. A minority of our advisory panel felt that the figure used was too low.

SUPPLY OF OPTOMETRISTS

Our projection model for optometrists is similar to the one for ophthalmologists. In the absence of AOA participation, data on optometrists and optometric practice patterns were more difficult to obtain. The AOA stated that it does not maintain a computerized or central membership database of member or non-member optometrists. We reviewed the optometric literature and made several assumptions about their number and their capabilities to treat eye disease. This section combines discussion of background information from that review with the final assumptions we made about optometrists before including them in our projection of future provider supply.

Number of Optometrists

Over 30,500 optometrists are licensed in the United States, and 27,000 are in practice (AOA, 1993). Seventy percent of optometrists are in private practice; 17.8 percent are employed by chains and superstores; 6.7 percent are employed by HMOs, hospitals, and clinics; 3.9 percent are in ophthalmologists' offices; and 1.7 percent are in the armed forces (AOA, 1993). The median age of practicing optometrists is 40 years (AOA, 1993).

In the contemporary health care market, optometrists have diagnostic privileges in all states, and 40 states extend therapeutic privileges to optometrists after certification. Table 3.5 displays the number of optometrists by type of practice privilege--diagnostic drug or therapeutic drug. The data in the table come from a variety of sources: American Academy of Ophthalmology, American Optometric Association, and the Census Bureau. As shown in the table, the number of optometrists in a state may be less than the number of certified optometrists. This is due to the fact that an individual optometrist may have more than one certification (DPA and TPA), and may additionally be certified in more than one state. Another source of information for the current number and distribution of licensed optometrists is the "Blue Book" of optometrists (1993). However, we did not use this data source because the AOA believes the book has substantial undercoverage problems.

Table 3.5
Distribution of Optometrists by State and Type of Privileges

State	Year DIAG/THER Laws Passed (1)	Total ODs (2)	Certi-fied ODs (1991) (3)	Type of Certification (%)		
				TPA	DPA	None
Alabama		349	466	0.0	100.0	0.0
Alaska	1988/1992	49	72	0.0	68.1	31.9
Arizona	1980/1993	425	540	0.0	56.9	43.1
Arkansas	1979/1987	348	289	72.7	8.3	19.0
California	1976	4,647	6,852	0.0	89.0	11.0
Colorado	1983/1988	612	758	53.8	18.9	27.3
Connecticut	1986/1992	442	697	0.0	61.0	39.0
Delaware	1975	22	90	0.0	100.0	0.0
D.C.	1986	0	310	0.0	22.3	77.7
Florida	1986/1986	1,342	1,722	67.2	0.0	32.8
Georgia	1980/1988	340	0	--	--	--
Hawaii	1985	287	173	0.0	87.9	12.1
Idaho	1981/1987	244	270	51.1	26.3	22.6
Illinois	1984	1,545	1,875	0.0	48.9	51.1
Indiana		1,035	1,004	0.0	0.0	100.0
Iowa	1979/1985	303	442	86.4	13.6	0.0
Kansas	1977/1987	386	438	70.1	15.8	14.1
Kentucky	1978/1986	300	560	63.8	17.0	19.2
Louisiana	1975/1993	459	451	0.0	0.0	100.0
Maine	1975/1987	115	183	72.1	7.1	20.8
Maryland	1989	558	566	0.0	56.7	43.3
Massachusetts	1985	923	1,585	0.0	28.3	71.7
Michigan	1984	1,115	1,052	0.0	63.2	36.8
Minnesota	1982/1993	417	763	0.0	61.7	38.3
Mississippi	1982	252	248	0.0	80.6	19.4
Missouri	1981/1986	775	828	55.7	12.2	32.1
Montana	1977/1987	285	274	36.1	63.9	0.0
Nebraska	1979/1986	148	234	65.4	17.9	16.7
Nevada	1979	156	160	0.0	92.5	7.5
New Hampshire	1985/1993	38	148	0.0	86.5	13.5
New Jersey	1992	1,181	1,092	0.0	100.0	0.0
New Mexico	1977/1985	345	219	51.6	48.4	0.0
New York	1983	1,922	2,369	0.0	56.5	43.5

Note: Table continues on next page.

Table 3.5
Distribution of Optometrists by State and Type of Privileges (continued)

State	Year DIAG/THER Laws Passed (1)	Total ODs (2)	Certi- fied ODs (1991) (3)	Type of Certification (%)		
				TPA	DPA	None
N. Carolina	1977/1977	618	755	88.2	0.0	11.8
North Dakota	1979/1987	95	178	65.7	15.7	18.6
Ohio	1984/1992	1,431	1,401	0.0	94.3	5.7
Oklahoma	1981/1984	375	558	75.4	0.0	24.6
Oregon	1975/1991	368	446	0.0	90.1	9.9
Pennsylvania	1974	1,411	2,544	0.0	81.0	19.0
Rhode Island	1971/1985	115	168	60.7	0.0	39.3
S. Carolina	1984/1993	330	240	0.0	41.3	58.7
South Dakota	1979/1986	207	136	62.5	22.1	15.4
Tennessee	1975/1987	519	1,040	38.5	0.0	61.5
Texas	1981/1991	1,759	1,673	0.0	36.5	63.5
Utah	1979/1991	154	273	0.0	100.0	0.0
Vermont	1984	15	121	0.0	52.1	47.9
Virginia	1983/1988	636	1,097	1.4	84.6	14.0
Washington	1981/1989	588	1,052	50.9	9.6	39.5
West Virginia	1976/1976	188	326	61.3	0.0	38.7
Wisconsin	1978/1989	584	1,218	30.1	45.4	24.5
Wyoming	1977/1987	126	106	76.4	3.8	19.8
Total		30,884	40,062	17.2	51.8	31.0

Sources: Information compiled from state licensing boards of optometry, except for (1) American Optometric Association, (2) Public-Use Micro Sample data, Bureau of the Census, 1990, and (3) American Academy of Ophthalmology.

NOTES: OD = Doctor of Optometry; TPA = therapeutic drug privilege; DPA = diagnostic drug privilege; THER = therapeutic; DIAG = diagnostic.

We were interested in estimating the number of certified optometrists by age and by location. Applying the percentages of optometrists with diagnostic drug privileges (DPA) or therapeutic drug privileges (TPA) to the total number of optometrists (ODs) in a state, we obtained a total of 27,664 certified optometrists, which is consistent with the estimate of 27,000 in practice (AOA, 1992). This is less than the 30,884 estimate derived from the census, which counts all people who call themselves "optometrists." We chose the lower figure because the AOA believes that this figure is more accurate. However, we do use the census data to provide age and gender distributions, because it is the only source of this information.

The data above suggest that about one-quarter of optometrists have therapeutic drug privileges and three-quarters have diagnostic drug privileges. However, this split is somewhat misleading because the legislative information is more current than the data on the number of optometrists. If we look at the number of optometrists in those states that had passed therapeutic privileges by 1990 (because our data on the number of optometrists is from 1991), we see that when therapeutic privileges are available, over half of the optometrists in the state seek therapeutic certification. From discussions with the AOA, we estimated that at this time, 50 percent of the certified optometrists are TPA-certified in states which passed TPA legislation, and we assumed that this number will rise to 100 percent by the year 2010. We also assumed that the current percentages of optometrists with TPA privileges vary differentially with age, according to the following schedule: (age<27: %TPA=100), (age=28-45: %TPA=50), (age=46-59: %TPA=40), (age=60-75: %TPA=30). This distribution assumes that all recent graduates are TPA-certified or certifiable and yields totals that approximate currently known DPA/TPA proportions.

Inflow

There are 17 accredited colleges of optometry in the United States and Puerto Rico; they graduated over 1,100 students in 1992-1993 (see Table 3.6). The majority (76.7 percent) of graduates are white, and half are male. The vast majority (98.5 percent) of recent graduates find positions in the optometric profession (ASCO, 1993). While there might be variation in the curriculum among schools, the trend in optometric education parallels the trends in licensure. Optometric training has increased its emphasis on training optometrists in the use of therapeutic pharmacological agents and other treatment modalities.

Table 3.6
1992-1993 U.S. Optometry School Graduates by Race and Gender

Race	Total	Percent Male	Race	Total	Percent Male
African American	68	21	Asian	147	29
Hispanic	44	57	Foreign	39	59
White	877	54	Other	8	75
			Total	1,143	51

Source: Association of Schools and Colleges of Optometry, 1993.

For example, we reviewed the catalog for the Southern California College of Optometry (SCCO, 1993). Starting in fall 1990, the SCCO required that all entrants complete at least three years of undergraduate college study before commencing optometric training. The optometric educational program at SCCO extends over four years, culminating in the doctorate of optometry degree. The first year of optometric training consists of courses related to the basic sciences and research techniques. The second year curriculum concerns clinical techniques and advanced courses in visual science. The third and fourth years consist of patient care activities, with some specialization occurring in the fourth year.

Outflow

Little is known specifically about the retirement and mortality (*outflow*) patterns experienced by optometrists. In the aggregate, approximately 600 optometrists leave the profession each year because of death or retirement (AOA, 1993). Using the Census Bureau's Public-Use Microdata Sample (PUMS), we created a synthetic age distribution that allowed us to apply the retirement and mortality rates to estimate the outflow of optometrists. We projected retirement and death for optometrists as we did for ophthalmologists, using the BHPr life table in the absence of optometry-specific rates. For 1994, using these life tables we estimated that approximately 600 optometrists will leave practice through retirement or death, which is similar to the number recently published by the AOA (Bennett and Aron, 1993).

Capacity

National surveys of health care use often do not include optometrists as providers. The National Ambulatory Medical Care Study surveys physician offices; optometrists are not included. The National Hospital Discharge Survey data set includes hospital discharges; provider information is not explicitly included, and the implicit assumption is that the primary care provider is a physician. These two sources of information, crucial to our understanding of the delivery of eye care services by physicians in ambulatory and hospital settings, did not assist us in estimating the contribution of optometry to eye care services.

Because we lack hard data to tell us otherwise, we assume that both ophthalmologists and optometrists spend the same amount of time treating patients with similar conditions. In addition, we assume that ophthalmologists and optometrists work the same number of hours per week and the same number of weeks per year. Thus, an optometric FTE is equivalent in time to an ophthalmologist FTE; that is, 2,016 hours per year. Again, the use of the FTE metric does not imply equivalence in quality, cost, or effectiveness of care, only in how long it takes to provide care and how long a provider works each year.

To be disease-specific, our model requires information about provider supply and capacity. Thus, we had to generate a list of diseases that we felt optometrists could treat. Moreover, we wanted to generate the lists by practice privilege type, that is, develop diagnostic- and therapeutic-privilege disease-specific lists. However, the fluidity in the current legislative processes concerning optometric privileges caused us not to consider the state-level variation but to develop a generalized list that broadly characterizes these two types of privilege-specific optometric practices.[7] Wherever doubt existed, it was resolved in favor of allowing optometrists to participate in the care of patients. Optometrists were excluded from the disease-specific

_____

[7]In the GMENAC study, optometrists were considered part of the eye care team, although specific conditions for which they provided care were not explicitly detailed except refractive errors, strabismus, and amblyopia.

provider supply only when the routine care of patients required systemic medical care or medications specifically excluded by law from optometric practice, or for surgery and surgical care. Given the net effect of all of these assumptions, we may overestimate the types of services provided by optometrists, which will result in an underestimate of any surplus of optometry providers (as well as of ophthalmology providers).

Final Assumptions

We are limited in what we know about optometrists' contributions to the provision of eye care services. These limitations are the result of the lack of data about the issues addressed by this workforce study. Certainly, we can model optometrists' provision of standard primary eye care, such as refractions, and we can vary this contribution to address, for example, proposals that optometrists provide all refractive services. However, many questions remain about the types of other services optometrists may provide, both diagnostic and therapeutic. Our approach was to maximize what optometrists could do in providing eye care services, because the AOA indicated that the trend was for states to adopt therapeutic drug regulations. To summarize the findings from the literature and special studies that shed light on optometric practice, we have listed the various assumptions (and constraints) we used in our models.

1. We had current (1991) state-level estimates of optometrists (Table 3.5, above) by type of certification (DPA or TPA).
2. We did not have the overall age and gender distribution of optometrists. We created a synthetic age and gender distribution using the PUMS data to obtain the distribution of optometrists by race and gender within each state. This distribution is important for aging the stock of optometrists and determining the annual outflow from the profession.
3. We knew the inflow of optometrists, i.e., the number of optometry graduates, into the market. We assumed they will distribute across states and counties according to historical patterns from the census. We also assumed that all new

optometrists will have the training to pass therapeutic-privilege examinations.

4. We assumed that optometry training extends over four years, with clinical activity occurring in years three and four. We assumed that third-year students provide the work equivalent of 35 percent of a fully licensed TPA optometrist FTE, and fourth-year students provide 50 percent of an FTE.[8] These figures are chosen to parallel those of ophthalmologist training, under the assumption that, in the absence of additional published data, the last two years of optometric training are clinically oriented. However, to the extent that clinical training differs between ophthalmology and optometry, the ratios may need to be adjusted.

5. We assumed that all states will pass optometrist therapeutic privilege statutes by the year 2010, and that the transition will be smooth: All new entrants will have TPA privileges, and a constant fraction will convert from DPA to TPA status.

6. We used information from Oklahoma (Walls et al., 1993) (a state in which optometrists have broader therapeutic drug privileges than in other states), various state statutes, and ophthalmologists' judgments to provide an inventory of the types of eye diseases that optometrists treat for the general population. This information is summarized in Table 3.7.

7. As we did for female ophthalmologists, we assumed that female optometrists provide 85 percent of an FTE.

8. We had no data on academic optometrists, so were unable to estimate their potential FTE contribution to the workforce.

---

[8]GMENAC did not include the contribution of optometry students in their analysis.

Table 3.7
Types of Diseases Treated by Optometrists, by Disease Group

Disease	DPA	TPA	Disease	DPA	TPA	Disease	DPA	TPA	Disease	DPA	TPA
01a	yes	yes	06a	yes	yes	09i	no	yes	11u	no	no
01b	no	yes	06b	yes	yes	09j	no	yes	12a	yes	yes
01c	no	yes	06c	yes	yes	10a	yes	yes	12b	yes	yes
01d	yes	yes	06d	yes	yes	10b	yes	yes	12c	yes	yes
02a	no	yes	07a	yes	yes	10c	yes	yes	12d	yes	yes
02b	no	yes	07b	yes	yes	11a	yes	yes	12e	yes	yes
02c	yes	yes	07c	yes	yes	11b	yes	yes	13a	no	yes
03a	no	yes	07d	no	no	11c	no	no	13b	no	yes
03b	no	yes	07e	no	no	11d	yes	yes	13c	no	no
03c	no	yes	07f	no	yes	11e	yes	yes	13d	no	no
03d	no	yes	07g	yes	yes	11f	yes	yes	13e	no	no
03e	no	yes	07h	yes	yes	11g	yes	yes	13f	no	no
03f	no	yes	08a	yes	yes	11h	yes	yes	13g	no	no
04a	no	yes	08b	no	no	11i	no	no	13h	no	no
04b	yes	yes	08c	no	no	11j	yes	yes	14a	no	no
04c	no	yes	08d	no	no	11k	no	no	14b	no	no
04d	no	yes	08e	no	no	11l	no	no	14c	no	no
04e	no	yes	09a	no	no	11m	no	yes	15a	no	yes
04f	no	yes	09b	no	no	11n	yes	yes	15b	no	yes
04g	no	yes	09c	yes	yes	11o	yes	yes	15c	no	yes
05a	no	yes	09d	no	yes	11p	yes	yes	15d	no	no
05b	yes	yes	09e	yes	yes	11q	no	no	15e	yes	yes
05c	no	yes	09f	yes	yes	11r	no	no	cont	yes	yes
05d	no	yes	09g	yes	yes	11s	yes	yes	refr	no	no
05e	no	yes	09h	no	no	11t	no	no	prev	yes	yes

NOTES: For definitions of diseases 01a through 15e, see Table 2.5.
Additional codes: cont=contact lens, refr = refractive surgery,
prev=preventive; TPA=therapeutic drug privileges; DPA=diagnostic
drug privileges.

Table 3.8
Projected Number of Optometrists: 1994-2010

	Beginning-of-Year Status			End-of-Year Status		
Year	Full	In-Training	FTE Optom.	Full	In-Training Graduates	Total Optom.
1994	27,510	2,000	27,646	26,910	997	27,907
1995	27,907	1,997	27,974	27,294	993	28,287
1996	28,287	1,997	28,287	27,662	993	28,655
1997	28,655	1,997	28,589	28,032	993	29,025
1998	29,025	1,997	28,892	28,412	993	29,405
1999	29,405	1,997	29,206	28,802	993	29,795
2000	29,796	1,997	29,531	29,209	993	30,202
2001	30,202	1,997	29,873	29,626	993	30,619
2002	30,619	1,997	30,224	30,065	993	31,058
2003	31,058	1,997	30,596	30,511	993	31,504
2004	31,504	1,997	30,978	30,974	993	31,967
2005	31,967	1,997	31,374	31,437	993	32,430
2006	32,430	1,997	31,772	31,921	993	32,914
2007	32,914	1,997	32,190	32,405	993	33,398
2008	33,398	1,997	32,610	32,911	993	33,904
2009	33,904	1,997	33,051	33,414	993	34,407
2010	34,408	1,997	33,492	33,921	993	34,914

Projecting the Supply of Optometrists

The projections of optometrists and the number of FTEs they provide during the years 1994 through 2010 (shown in Table 3.8) are done in a series of five steps in a manner similar to that for ophthalmologists:

1. At the beginning of a year, we counted the number of optometrists and optometrist trainees, taking care to allocate only a fraction of the third- and fourth-year trainees to the FTE work supply.

2. During the year, optometrists die and retire at age- and gender-specific rates. These rates were drawn from the BHPr (Greenberg, 1992).

3. Fourth-year trainees graduate and become full-fledged TPA optometrists in the following year.

4. Third-year optometry trainees are registered into their first clinical year. For all years, we assumed an entering cohort of 1,000 optometrists, which approximately matches historical rates of entry. We assumed all will become TPA optometrists.

5. We iterated these steps out to the year 2010.

OTHER PHYSICIAN SUPPLY

Many eye conditions and diseases can be diagnosed and treated by
other physicians. Examples include conjunctivitis, corneal abrasions,
dry eye, blowout fractures, ptosis repair, and other external diseases.
Other conditions that can be treated by nonophthalmologist physicians
(e.g., neurosurgeons) include systemic diseases with eye or ocular
manifestations, such as cranial nerve abnormalities, occipital lobe
strokes, and other neurological or orbital problems. To better describe
this situation, we analyzed the NAMCS database to determine the
frequency with which diagnoses are made, by type of physician. We
identified a set of diseases for which physicians other than
ophthalmologists provided at least 15 percent of the volume of care
that ophthalmologists provided (as measured by the number of visits).
We then excluded those conditions for which ophthalmic training was
required for quality care (e.g., intraocular conditions) to arrive at a
set of conditions for which other physicians were eligible to treat
(medically or surgically). For example, a non-ophthalmologist diagnosis
of endophthalmitis, glaucoma, or corneal dystrophy is excluded because
non-ophthalmologists do not treat or follow such conditions. Table 3.9
identifies the diseases and provides the percentage treated by non-
ophthalmologist physicians, according to the NAMCS database.

Because there is no reason to expect that these treatment patterns
will decrease, we included this pool of providers by adjusting the
disease-specific required FTEs downward in proportion to the level of
care provided by the other physicians, as reflected in the NAMCS data
set. As noted above, concerns about data accuracy of diagnostic coding
and physician subspecialty designation limited us to making this
adjustment only for those conditions in which nonophthalmologist
physicians provided at least 15 percent of the visits.

The inclusion of nonophthalmologist physicians will reduce the
number of FTE eye care providers required to treat a given disease. We
used refined methods (i.e., linear programming) to allocate only
optometrists and ophthalmologists and not nonophthalmologist physicians

because the need or demand for care by for non-eye-care services could not be separately estimated for these providers. These physicians provide a wide range of other services not included in our survey; there was no basis for providing an estimate of the relative priorities for these services. Thus, nonophthalmologist physicians could not be included in the linear programming for allocation of patient care among eye care providers.

Table 3.9
Proportion of Eye Care Diseases Treated by
Non-Ophthalmologist Physicians, By Disease Group

Disease	Percentage Non-ophthalmologist	Disease	Percentage Non-ophthalmologist
02a	78.0	08a	46.5
02b	60.8	08b	85.0
02c	29.9	09a	32.9
04c	29.2	09b	30.6
04e	19.2	09c	74.5
07b	46.6	09d	23.9
07c	52.8	13a	51.7
07d	88.4	13b	41.4
07e	20.1	13d	72.2
07f	51.7		

Source: National Ambulatory Medical Care Survey, 1989, 1990, 1991. See Table 2.5 for the condition corresponding to the number.

Given the much larger pool of nonophthalmologist physicians, even when limited to the appropriate subspecialties for each of the conditions in question (e.g, plastic surgery and otolaryngology for blowout fractures), we assumed that the proportion of eye care derived from the past NAMCS practices will continue and will be met by the available pool of nonophthalmologist physicians. Indeed, given the financial exigencies of capitation and managed care, the proportion of eye care delivered by primary care and other physicians might actually increase instead of decrease. Conversely, subcapitation by specialists such as ophthalmologists may increase the proportion of eye care services delivered by eye care providers, because general physicians would then not be financially at risk. Therefore, we use the NAMCS proportions as the base estimate. Alternative modeling could be conducted using some of these assumptions, but it was not explored in this study.

SUMMARY

This model estimates the supply of ophthalmologists and optometrists as the primary providers of eye care services. Other physicians are included because they provide a significant amount of eye care treatment for certain conditions. Other professional staff also contribute to the provision of eye care services in the United States, for example, opticians, certified ophthalmic technicians, ophthalmic registered nurses, etc. However, such providers were not included in our analysis of provider supply because they cannot provide services independently.

The results of our workforce supply projections show that the supply of ophthalmologists and optometrists will continue to grow through the year 2010. If current training patterns persist, the supply of FTE ophthalmologists will grow 11 percent and the supply of FTE optometrists will grow 24 percent (the difference in the supply growth is a reflection of the younger average age of optometrists). Further, our model assumes that optometrists in training today and in the future will gain therapeutic drug certification.

4. NEED AND DEMAND FOR EYE CARE PROVIDERS

Estimates of workforce requirements have traditionally been based on extrapolations from current utilization patterns (*demand*). Yet many lay and professional organizations focus on a particular disease or condition and estimate the number of people with those specific conditions, whether or not they have been treated (*need*). Population-based, methodologically sound epidemiological studies of the true incidence and prevalence of specific diseases (*true need*) are generally lacking. Because there can be significant differences in the number of people afflicted and the number of people who actually receive care, this study provides workforce estimates based on separate models of need and demand so that direct comparison to demand estimates used in contemporary workforce estimates can be made and additional information on the workforce required to fully or otherwise better meet public health need can be modeled.

The basis for developing separate models can be found in contemporary health services research findings. For example, it is estimated that only half of those with diabetes currently realize they have diabetes and would benefit from a physician's care (Prevent Blindness America, 1994). Also, the poor are less likely to receive the care they need for a wide range of medical conditions. To establish workforce requirements based solely on current utilization patterns (demand) would lock in place current inequities in care provision as well as current patterns of providing care.

At the same time, there is a dearth of studies on population incidence and prevalence of various medical and ocular conditions. Where such studies are available, they form the basis of the need model for those specific conditions or diseases. Population-based and other studies are available for conditions that constitute about 60 percent of current, problem-oriented utilization, (i.e., doctor visits or hospitalizations) and would constitute over 85% of need. Thus, we were able to compare the level of demand for eye care services with the estimated true public health need. Where no such studies were available, we rescaled current disease-specific demand rates by the need-to-demand ratio for related diseases. Where such rescaling seemed inappropriate (e.g., trauma cases), we took the conservative approach of utilizing current demand rates.

In both models--need and demand--we estimated the number of individuals with a given condition or disease, based on scientific studies (need) or current utilization, as reflected in the NAMCS data set (primarily) and the NHDS.

Our goal is to estimate need and demand for FTE eye care providers. In Chapter Two we reviewed the incidence and prevalence information and population data available for this task. The remaining required piece of information is work-time estimates. In this chapter, we describe how we processed the survey-based work-time data to obtain work-time estimates for the 97 disease groupings for the medical and surgical components of care. Then we describe our algorithm for combining these data. Finally, we present the results for the 15 aggregate disease and rehabilitation categories.

CLINICAL NEED

As discussed in Chapter Two, we used incidence and prevalence rates to estimate the public health need for eye care services from a variety of sources. We used rates derived from major population-based epidemiological studies for the leading causes of visual impairment in the United States: cataract, glaucoma, macular degeneration, diabetic retinopathy, and myopia. Information on incidence and prevalence rates for other conditions, such as other forms of refractive error, strabismus, choroidal tumors, and trauma, were obtained from recognized national databases, such as those reported in *Vital and Health Statistics*. (See Table 2.6). Other data were obtained from published reports in the scientific literature, such as the rates of some neuro-ophthalmological conditions, color blindness, or congenital cataracts. Finally, where no other sources of information were available, we used demand rates from the National Ambulatory Medical Care Survey (NAMCS) and the National Hospital Discharge Survey (NHDS). We rescaled these demand-based data to need, using need-to-demand ratios derived from other comparable disease groupings that had such information available.

Using these disease-/condition-specific incidence and prevalence rates, we calculated the population of individuals who are affected by each disease or condition. However, as noted in Chapter Two, not every individual who has a condition requires care at a level above that of periodic monitoring during preventive health visits. Thus, with the assistance of the advisory panel and other ophthalmologists, we created clinical population fractional multipliers to adjust the affected population to a *clinical population*, which we define as persons needing specific care for their disease or condition. Where no solid data or evidence exist to justify such a modification, the affected population is not adjusted and is counted fully as the clinical population. The resulting estimated clinical population is the base to which provider work times are applied to derive the number of FTEs required for eye care.

PROVIDER WORK TIMES

To calculate the workforce required to provide eye care services, it is necessary to know the time required to care for a given condition or disease in a year. The RAND Eye Care Workforce Survey (RWS) gathered data on these times for most of the 97 disease and rehabilitation groupings from a survey of ophthalmologists. We distinguish between medical (office) and surgical time, and describe our methods for estimating these quantities below.

Office Visit Times

Each type of ophthalmic subspecialist and general ophthalmologist received a questionnaire with questions about typical diagnoses for that subspecialty. Figures 4.1 and 4.2 show the tables that we requested cornea subspecialists to fill out. Answers to survey questions provided information on the length of initial visit, the number of follow-up

Section 3: MEDICAL VISITS

Please complete the following table providing information concerning your **typical** patient. We are interested in obtaining data which reflect your experience in your practice. That is, provide the information only for those diagnoses you see in your practice and for which you feel comfortable providing estimates.

INITIAL VISITS

For example, in your practice you saw 10 new cataract patients in the last 30 days. The initial evaluation takes on average 35 minutes which is comprised of 20 minutes of your time, 5 minutes of technician's time, and 10 minutes of optometrist's time.

DIAGNOSIS	Your Practice (A) Estimate of **Number** of **NEW** patients seen in the last 30 days	Ophthalmologist Average length of **INITIAL** visit in minutes	Optometrist Average length of **INITIAL** visit in minutes	Registered Nurse Average length of **INITIAL** visit in minutes	Technician/ Technologist Average length of **INITIAL** visit in minutes
Cataract	10	20	10	0	5
CORNEAL INFECTION					
SUPERFICIAL FOREIGN BODY					
DRY EYE					
CORNEAL DYSTROPHY					
CORNEAL EDEMA					
PTERYGIUM					
CORNEAL OPACITY					
CORNEAL DEPOSITS					

Fig. 4.1--RAND Eye Care Workforce Survey: Initial Medical Visits

FOLLOW-UP MEDICAL VISITS

For example, your typical cataract patient may make 4 follow-up visits each year to your office. You see the patient on 3 of these visits and they typically require 20 minutes of your time and 5 minutes of nurse time. In addition, your typical cataract patients may visit the optometrist once in your office during the year for a 30 minute visit. Finally, you estimate that 30 percent of your cataract patients proceed to incisional surgery each year and none proceed to laser surgery.

DIAGNOSIS	Your Practice (B) — Estimate of Number of follow-up patients seen in last 30 days	Ophthalmologist — Average Number of Follow-up visits per year	Ophthalmologist — Average length of Follow-up visits in minutes	Optometrist — Average Number of Follow-up visits per year	Optometrist — Average length of Follow-up visits in minutes	Registered Nurse — Average Number of Follow-up visits per year	Registered Nurse — Average length of Follow-up visits in minutes	Technician/Technologist — Average Number of Follow-up visits per year	Technician/Technologist — Average length of Follow-up visits in minutes	Your Practice (C) — Percent of patients who proceed to surgery: Laser	Your Practice (C) — Percent of patients who proceed to surgery: Incisional
Cataract	4	4	20	1	30	3	5	0	0	0 %	30 %
CORNEAL INFECTION										%	%
SUPERFICIAL FOREIGN BODY										%	%
DRY EYE										%	%
CORNEAL DYSTROPHY										%	%
CORNEAL EDEMA										%	%
PTERYGIUM										%	%
CORNEAL OPACITY										%	%
CORNEAL DEPOSITS										%	%

Fig. 4.2--RAND Eye Care Workforce Survey: Follow-up Visits

visits per year, and the average length of time for follow-up visits. Figure 4.2 also shows that the survey requested information on the rates at which patients with a given disease undergo procedures (laser or incisional) in a given year.

Surgery Times (Laser and Incisional)

In the RWS, members of each subspecialty category were given a list of common procedures in their subspecialty area. The particular variables of interest were physician pre-operative assessment times, intra-operative time by a surgeon, other same-day operative time by a surgeon, and the number and length of post-operative visits. As an example, Figures 4.3 and 4.4 show the tables that we used to request the surgical information from cornea specialists.

Survey Data Time Estimates

We assembled these survey data, then aggregated them up to the 97 disease groupings. The results of the aggregation are shown in Tables 4.1 and 4.2. There were five steps in this aggregation.

1. Relate each survey entry to one or more of the 97 groupings. For diagnoses (Figures 4.1 and 4.2), the mapping is 1:1. For procedures (Figures 4.3 and 4.4), the mapping is one-to-many: that is, a given procedure may be applied to several different disease groupings.

2. For each of the 97 disease groupings, assemble all related responses from Step 1, regardless of the subspecialty category of the respondent and regardless of whether the particular item is a procedure that relates to other diseases as well.

Section 4: SURGICAL TIME REQUIREMENTS

Please complete table by filling in the times for those procedures that you do. We are interested in getting numbers that reflect your practice patterns. Please provide information for those procedures that you personally perform and for which you are comfortable providing estimates.

PRE-OPERATIVE ASSESSMENT AND INTRA-OPERATIVE TIME

For example, in the last 30 days you performed 2 trabeculectomies. In your practice a typical trabeculectomy requires 60 minutes of pre-operative assessment by the ophthalmologist, 10 minutes of a nurse and 20 minutes of an ophthalmic technician. The surgery (skin-to-skin) takes 45 minutes of surgeon time and 55 minutes of nurse time. Other Operative time includes 20 minutes each of the surgeon and the nurse for dictation, talking to the family, and other activities.

		Time in minutes for typical patient									
	Your Practice	Pre-operative Assessment				Intra-operation Time (skin-to-skin)			Other Operative Time (same day, including dictation)		
NAME OF PROCEDURE	Estimate of number of patients operated on in the last 30 days	MD	Optometrist	RN	Tech	Surgeon	RN	Tech	Surgeon	RN	Tech
		(min)	(min)	(min)	(min)	(min)	(min)	(min)	(min)	(min)	(min)
Trabeculectomy	2	60	0	10	20	45	55	0	20	20	0
CORNEAL TRANSPLANT											
PTERYGIUM EXCISION											
REMOVE CORNEAL EPITHELIUM											
CORNEAL BIOPSY											

Fig. 4.3--RAND Eye Care Workforce Survey: Pre-Operative Assessment and Intra-Operative Time

POST-OPERATIVE PERIOD (90 DAYS POST SURGERY)

For example, in the period immediately following surgery (that is, 90 days post-op), you may see the typical patient 10 times for 10 minutes each visit. During all visits, the technician spends 5 minutes with the patient. The optometrist sees the patient twice for 15 minutes each visit, and the nurse sees the typical trabeculectomy patient 3 times for 5 minutes per visit.

NAME OF PROCEDURE	Ophthalmologist		Optometrist		Registered Nurse		Technician/ Technologist	
	# of visits in 90 days	Avg. visit time in minutes	# of visits in 90 days	Avg. visit time in minutes	# of visits in 90 days	Avg. visit time in minutes	# of visits in 90 days	Avg. visit time in minutes
Trabeculectomy	10	10	2	15	3	5	10	5
CORNEAL TRANSPLANT								
PTERYGIUM EXCISION								
REMOVE CORNEAL EPITHELIUM								
CORNEAL BIOPSY								
REFRACTIVE KERATOTOMY								
EXCIMER PRK								

Fig. 4.4--RAND Eye Care Workforce Survey: Post-Operative Period

3. Aggregate numbers of visits and visit times for each disease grouping using unweighted averages and medians, respectively.[9]

4. For percentages (e.g., proportion proceeding to surgery), compute unweighted averages. Means, rather than medians, were used here because these data were fairly unsymmetric. In general, there were many zeroes in the percentages of patients proceeding to surgery, and the median rates to surgery were often lower than our advisory panel thought was appropriate.

5. For disease groupings not covered by the questionnaire items, use estimates from a similar disease grouping. Out of 97 groupings, this was done for 17 disease groupings for office activity, 24 for incisional procedure times, and 19 for laser procedure times. These accounted for less than 5 percent of patients altogether.

Tables 4.1 and 4.2 show the types of results that went into our analysis. *Office activity* is described by the length and frequency of initial and follow-up visits and by the percentage of patients who proceed to surgery. *Surgical activity* is described by the actual amount of surgical time, plus pre- and post-operative visits. For presentation purposes, the results are given here only for the first and last few disease or condition groupings. Appendix B contains the full tables.

_____

[9]The decision to use medians was based on the distribution of the data, which revealed that the data were fairly symmetric about their central value, but included a few outliers on the low and high ends. Medians and means both estimate the center of a symmetric distribution, but medians are much less sensitive to outliers than means. The decision to do unweighted computations was implied by our sample design. To get information for the 97 disease groupings, we generally had to limit questions about each disease to a single subspecialty; within subspecialty groups, the sampling weights were equal, because we stratified on subspecialty in drawing our samples. To check whether the assumption of equal weights introduced bias in the population of responding ophthalmologists, we examined differences between the full and responding populations, and estimated the effects of these differences on our projections; these effects are discussed in the robustness section of Chapter Five.

Table 4.1
Components of Office Work Time

| | | Office Time | | | Percentage Proceeding to Surgery | |
| | | Initial Visit | Follow-up Visits | | | |
Disease	Description	Time (min)	Freq	Time (min)	Laser	Incision
01a	cataract	20	2	15	0	30
01b	lens-related diseases	20	2	15	0	9
01c	aphakia / pseudophakia	20	1	15	13	1
01d	congenital cataract	30	2	15	4	12
.	.	.	.	.	.	.
.	.	.	.	.	.	.
15a	herpes simplex	25	5	15	2	7
15b	herpes zoster	30	4	15	4	11
15c	iris lesions	30	2	20	3	15
15d	other ocular infections	30	5	15	0	61
15e	other	20	2	15	1	21

NOTE: For the full listing of this table, see Appendix B.

Table 4.2

Components of Incisional and Laser Surgical Times

Disease Group and Description	Incisional Surgical Time (minutes)			Post-op		Laser Surgical Times (minutes)			Post-op	
	Pre-Op	Intra-Op	Same Day	Freq	Time (min)	Pre-Op	Intra-Op	Same Day	Freq	Time (min)
01a cataract	30	40	20	5	12					
01b lens-related diseases	30	40	20	5	10					
01c aphakia / pseudophakia	30	35	15	4	10	20	10	5	2	10
01d congenital cataract	30	45	20	5	15					
.	.	.	.	.	.	.	.	.	.	.
.	.	.	.	.	.	.	.	.	.	.
15a herpes simplex	30	20	10	4	10	30	30	12	3	15
15b herpes zoster	30	20	10	4	10	30	20	10	3	15
15c iris lesions	45	60	20	10	12	30	15	10	4	10
15d other ocular infection	30	45	15	5	15	30	20	10	3	15
15e other	30	40	20	5	12					

NOTES: For the full listing of this table, see Appendix B. Op = operative time.

NEED AND DEMAND SPREADSHEET COMPUTATIONS

This section documents the computations performed to produce the need estimates. The data input to these computations are shown in Table 4.3. Included in this table are variable definitions as well as parameters estimated from the RWS data. The following subsections detail the computations.

Table 4.3
Variables For Need and Demand Spreadsheet Computations

Input Variable	Description
By age, race, and gender	
POP	population estimates (Chapter Two)
By 97 disease groupings	
PREVRATE	prevalence rates, by age, possibly race and gender (Chapter Two)
INCRATE	incidence rates, by age, possibly race and gender (Chapter Two)
FVOPH	number of follow-up visits to an ophthalmologist in a year (RWS)
FVLOPH	length of follow-up visit to an ophthalmologist (RWS)
IVLOPH	length of initial visit to an ophthalmologist (RWS)
PCTLASER	percentage proceeding to laser surgery (RWS)
PCTINC	percentage proceeding to incisional surgery (RWS)
PROBP	percentage of prevalent population needing clinical treatment (RWS)
PROBI	percentage of incident population needing clinical treatment (RWS)
PREMD	preoperative time by an ophthalmologist (RWS)
INTSURG	surgical time (skin-to-skin) by an ophthalmologist (RWS)
OTHSURG	other same-day time by an ophthalmologist (RWS)

Table 4.3
Variables For Need and Demand Spreadsheet Computations (continued)

Input Variable	Description
POSOPHV	number of post-operative visits by an ophthalmologist (RWS)
POSOPHT	length of post-operative visits (RWS)
OLDVIS	prevalent visits per year (NAMCS and NHDS; see Chapter Two)
NEWINC	incident visits per year (NAMCS and NHDS; see Chapter Two)
PCT1	percentage of visits with one chronic condition (NAMCS)
PCT2	percentage of visits with two chronic conditions (NAMCS)
PCT3	percentage of visits with three chronic conditions (NAMCS) *parameters*
FTE	2,016 = ophthalmologist work hours per year (Chapter Three)
MULTDSE	1.433 = average number of eye conditions for an individual with at least one eye condition (NAMCS)
PCT1	64.4 = percentage visits with one eye condition (NAMCS)
PCT2	27.9 = percentage visits with two eye conditions (NAMCS)
PCT3	7.7 = percentage visits with three eye conditions (NAMCS)
LEN1	17.1 = length of visits with one eye condition (NAMCS)
LEN2	17.7 = length of visits with two eye conditions (NAMCS)
LEN3	20.8 = length of visits with three eye conditions (NAMCS)

NOTES: Sources are shown in parentheses. RWS = RAND Eye Care Workforce Survey.

Differences in Computing Need Versus Demand

The only difference between the need and the demand calculations is in the number of persons with the given condition. For demand, this is the number of cases, or individuals, that are seen. For need, this is the number of cases that *should* be seen.

Demand. NAMCS gives us the number of visits, not cases. However, NAMCS does tell us whether a case is new (NEWINC), thus giving us incidence numbers. To estimate prevalence, we took the number of visits characterized as continuing care (OLDVIS), and divided by the number of follow-up visits (FVOPH) per year obtained from the survey. Thus,

$$INC\_DEMAND_i = NEWINC_i, \tag{4.1}$$

$$PREV\_DEMAND_i = OLDVIS_i/FVOPH_i \tag{4.2}$$

where the subscript i denotes one of the 97 disease groupings.

Need. We disaggregated the U.S. population into 400 demographic groups: 100 ages, 2 races (African-American, other), and 2 genders. Our population counts are 1990 census population estimates, and census projections to the years 2000 and 2010. For each of these demographic combinations, we applied the corresponding incidence and prevalence rates (sometimes available only by aggregate demographic groups) to estimate the number of persons with the given condition; then we aggregated these numbers over race, gender, and age to the 97 disease groupings:

$$POP\_INC_i = \sum_{r,g,a} [POP_{r,g,a} * INCRATE_{i,r,g,a}], \tag{4.3}$$

$$POP\_PREV_i = \sum_{r,g,a} [POP_{r,g,a} * PREVRATE_{i,r,g,a}], \tag{4.4}$$

where the subscript i=disease, r=race, g=gender, and a=age. We then converted these numbers to estimates of clinical incidence and prevalence, using our clinical population modifiers for prevalent (PROBP) and incident (PROBI) cases:

$$INC\_NEED_i = POP\_INC_i * PROBI_i \tag{4.5}$$

$$PREV\_NEED_i = POP\_PREV_i * PROBP_i \tag{4.6}$$

These 97 disease-specific estimates of need and demand were entered into the spreadsheet as (PREV_DEMAND,INC_DEMAND) or (PREV_NEED,INC_NEED). In the description below, we use the "NEED" suffix and drop the subscript i to simplify exposition.

Office Work Computations

Given the number of cases, we can compute the amounts of work by work type performed by eye care providers. All times are converted to FTEs by dividing by 60 (to convert minutes to hours), then dividing by 2,016 (our estimate of the number of patient contact hours provided by an FTE provider in a given year).

Initial visit (IWORK) and follow-up visit (FWORK) work times are computed as functions of the number of such visits (ivoph=1, FVOPH) and the length of visit (IVLOPH, FVLOPH):

$$IWORK = INC\_NEED * (IVLOPH+.5*FVOPH*FVLOPH) \qquad (4.7)$$

$$FWORK = PREV\_NEED * (FVOPH*FVLOPH) \qquad (4.8)$$

The second factor in IWORK reflects an assumption that, on average, the incident cases occur halfway through the year, so each new patient receives a half-year's worth of follow-up visits during the year of incidence.

These numbers, however, should be adjusted for multiple conditions. Patients may have more than one disease. In NAMCS, we found that the average number of eye conditions for a patient seeing an ophthalmologist was 1.433. Thus, many individuals may be counted twice or more in our incidence and prevalence estimates. We therefore adjusted for the fact that a patient with multiple conditions does not necessarily require separate visits for each condition or that the length of visits is not necessarily the mathematical sum of such visits.

The questions in the RAND Eye Care Workforce Survey concerning initial and follow-up office work were targeted to a single condition. From NAMCS, we estimated the percentage of time that one (PCT1), two (PCT2), or three (PCT3) different eye diseases occur, as well as the relative ratios of time necessary to treat one (LEN1), two (LEN2), or three (LEN3) diseases. We compiled the percentages by disease, but aggregated the ratios across all diseases because the average lengths of time in NAMCS by disease were too variable for different orderings of some combinations of diseases and no scientific data exist as to disease combinations aside from a few major conditions such as cataract, macular degeneration, diabetes and glaucoma. Applying these adjustments to the estimates of work derived above, we get

$$IWORK' = IWORK*(PCT1+ (LEN2/LEN1)*PCT2/2+ (LEN2/LEN1)*PCT3/3)/100 \quad (4.9)$$

$$FWORK' = FWORK*(PCT1+ (LEN2/LEN1)*PCT2/2+ (LEN3/LEN1)*PCT3/3)/100 \quad (4.10)$$

The logic of these formulas is as follows. One condition occurs PCT1 percent of the time; PCT1 therefore simply multiplies the unadjusted work level. Two conditions occur PCT2 percent of the time. A certain increase in visit time occurs because two conditions are present, which we estimate by the ratio (LEN2/LEN1). But that increase will be counted twice, once for each of the two conditions that the patient has. Thus, we divide by 2 to readjust this number, as seen in the second term in the composite multiplier. Similarly, three conditions occur PCT3 percent of the time, they take longer than a single disease by the ratio (LEN3/LEN1), and they are divided by three to avoid triple-counting, leading to the last term in the composite multiplier. This composite multiplier adjusts both for the patient with more than one disease and for the incremental length of time required to take care of patients with more than one disease.

To get total medical work, we simply add initial and follow-up visit times:

$$MEDWORK = IWORK' + FWORK' \quad (4.11)$$

Surgical Work Computations

The RWS recorded the components of surgical work times for various eye-related procedures. After estimating the aggregate median surgical time for each of these components, within disease grouping and by the laser or incisional nature of the procedure, these components were combined according to the following formulas:

Incisional procedures:

$$INCTIME = PREMD+INTSURG+OTHSURG+POSOPHV*POSOPHT \quad (4.12)$$

$$INCWORK = (PREV\_NEED+INC\_NEED)*(PCTINC /100)*INCTIME \quad (4.13)$$

Laser procedures:

$$LASTIME = PREMD+INTSURG+OTHSURG+POSOPHV*POSOPHT \qquad (4.14)$$

$$LASWORK = (PREV\_NEED+INC\_NEED)*(PCTLASER/100)*LASTIME \qquad (4.15)$$

To get total surgical work, we added the times associated with incisional and laser surgery:

$$SURGWORK = INCWORK + LASWORK. \qquad (4.16)$$

Preventive Services

Preventive services are clearly important forms of care, but they have not been captured in utilization surveys that are disease-treatment-oriented. We chose to adopt the preventive eye care schedule for those 18 years of age and younger developed by the March 1994 National Eye Care Forum Consensus Conference (see Table 2.4) and the AAO Preferred Practice Pattern for preventive services for adults (see Chapter 2). The schedule enabled us to estimate FTE requirements for preventive work.

We obtained our estimates of preventive work in four steps.

1. Tabulate the U.S. population by race and age.
2. Subtract from the U.S. population the estimated number of people, by race and age, who will receive clinical treatment for eye problems. We described earlier in this chapter how the clinical population is estimated from incidence and prevalence estimates and from clinical multipliers. To avoid double-counting persons with multiple eye problems, we divided the clinical population by the average number of eye conditions for an individual with at least one eye condition (MULTDSE, from Table 4.3), which gives us the estimates, by race and age, of persons not receiving problem-oriented care who are thus eligible for preventive eye care services.
3. Apply the preventive visit schedule to the population estimates obtained in Step 2. This gives us the recommended number of

preventive exams in a year: 45, 49, and 51 million for the years 1994, 2000, and 2010, respectively.

4. Convert preventive exam counts to FTE requirements by assuming preventive exams take 20 minutes each and are done by a professional who works the standard number of hours per year (FTE, from Table 4.3).

Elective Services

We decided to narrowly define elective services and include only those services for which some information is available: contact lens fitting and refractive surgery. Elective surgery and contact lens rates were estimated on the basis of summary figures obtained from subspecialty societies, the AOA, and eye care device manufacturers.

Contact Lenses. We attempted to estimate the amount of time separate from what was delivered in the course of routine care for disease grouping 10; that is, the amount of time spent dealing with contact lens problems. We began with the estimated total refractive error <u>clinical</u> population (38 million in 1994) and assumed that a certain fraction (50 percent) opts for contact lenses (19 million in the entire U.S. population). For the prevalent population, we assumed that 10 percent of the contact lens users develop problems each year that require an additional 15-minute visit. For the incident population, we assumed that 20 percent of the contact lens users develop problems that require an additional 15-minute visit. Using our estimate of standard work hours per year (FTE, from Table 4.3), we get 239 FTEs allocated to contact lens problems. We recognize that these numbers may appear low, but note that severe problems would be covered under the cornea and external disease groups.

Refractive Surgery. We started with the estimated myopic clinical and refractive error populations and treated prevalent and incident populations the same. We assumed that 1.5 percent of the clinical population opts for the surgery, and, from our survey, we estimated that the procedure takes a total of 110 minutes. Using our estimate of standard work hours per year (FTE, from Table 4.3) yielded 232 FTEs allocated to refractive surgery.

Spreadsheet Computation Results

Aggregate totals from the preceding computations are shown in Table 4.4. They are the disaggregated estimates of FTE requirements that will be matched with the supply numbers derived in Chapter Three.

Table 4.4
Final Estimates of Demand and Need from Spreadsheet

Disease	Need		Demand		Need (2000)		Need (2010)	
	Med	Surg	Med	Surg	Med	Surg	Med	Surg
01a	1,567	2,788	904	1,541	1,836	3,266	2,124	3,781
01b	1	0	1	0	1	0	1	0
01c	1,812	1,229	467	303	2,122	1,438	2,460	1,668
01d	9	6	3	2	9	6	9	6
.	.	.	.	.	.	.	.	
.	.	.	.	.	.	.	.	
15b	1	0	15	4	2	0	2	1
15c	13	8	9	6	13	9	14	10
15d	0	0	1	2	0	0	0	0
15e	58	74	30	37	62	79	65	84
Contact lens	239	0	239	0	257	0	270	0
Refractive surgery	0	232	0	232	0	250	0	263
Preventive	9,808	0	12,897	0	10,498	0	11,004	0
Total	23,808	7,611	19,069	4,003	26,242	8,705	28,430	9,843

NOTE: For the full listing of this table, see Appendix B.

Summary

The determination of the requirements for eye care providers can be based on meeting current utilization levels (demand) or upon meeting the needs for care of every person with a significant clinical condition (public health need). The kind of data needed, the precision with which such data are gathered, and the availability of such data vary between these two views of the workforce required for eye care. Data from current utilization databases, such as the National Ambulatory Medical Care Survey (NAMCS), the National Hospital Discharge Survey (NHDS), the National Health Interview Survey (NHIS), and the Medicare MEDPAR files were used to provide or confirm the accuracy of data for demand projections. Data for need estimates were obtained from several sources, starting with the Baltimore, Beaver Dam, and Framingham Eye Studies. Scientific publications and input from Prevent Blindness America were also used. These two types of sources provided prevalence or incidence data for conditions which currently account for approximately 60 percent of problem-oriented demand or utilization. Additional estimates for those conditions without such data sources were generated from scaling known demand estimates upwards by a factor calculated from a similar disease condition for which both need and demand were known. Finally, not all patients with a condition require medical care outside of that provided in a routine preventive visit; a clinical modifier was thus used to reduce the patient population for certain conditions.

RAND also conducted a workforce survey in order to determine the time required to care for eye conditions and diseases, as well as the need for laser or incisional surgery. The estimates were reviewed by the Advisory Panel and the surgical rates and numbers compared to known demand in the MEDPAR files. The time required to care for conditions was then combined with the clinical number of individuals with a given condition to determine the time required to provide eye care in a given year. The number of FTEs required was then calculated by including a work-year rate of 2,016 hours of direct patient care (exclusive of specific system-dependent requirements such as special prior approval forms or other similar issues).

The results of the analyses and models indicate that current demand for eye care requires 23,072 FTEs, and current need requires 31,419 FTEs. When care provided by other physicians is included (see Chapter Three), the FTEs demanded are 22,154 and the FTEs needed are 30,757. The reconciliation of supply with these two estimates of requirements occurs in the next chapter.

5. SUPPLY AND REQUIREMENTS RECONCILIATION

This chapter discusses the methods used to reconcile the supply estimates (from Chapter Three) with the requirements estimates (from Chapter Four). The purpose of this reconciliation is to answer three basic questions:

1. Are there enough eye care providers to serve the needs and demands of the U.S. population?
2. What kinds of combinations between optometrists and ophthalmologists are possible to meet the eye care needs of the U.S. population?
3. Are there enough subspecialists to meet surgical demand and need for care and treatment of eye diseases within their specialization?

We first describe our methods and then present results for four base cases: demand, current need, and projected need for the years 2000 and 2010. A final section of this chapter describes our efforts to assess the robustness of our models. We evaluate the stability of our findings against possible response biases in the RAND Eye Care Workforce Survey, examine variation in our results by census region, and look at errors due to uncertainties in our estimates of the numerous parameters that constitute the basis of our calculations.

RECONCILIATION METHODS

Problem Setup

We use linear programming techniques to perform the reconciliation. Our formulation attempts to allocate suppliers into the cells of a two-way matrix, where the rows index all eye-care-specific work categories and the columns identify FTE eye care providers (optometrists and ophthalmologists). Table 5.1 illustrates the format of the data table for reconciling need and supply. The leftmost column identifies 197 different classes of work: two (medical and surgical) for each of the 97

Table 5.1

Format of Data Table for Reconciliation Step

Grouping	CAT	COR	GEN	GLAU	LV	NEUR	PLAS	RET	STR	UV	DPA	TPA	Adjusted Need
01a Med													1,567
01a Surg													2,788
01b Med													1
01c Med													1,812
01c Surg													1,229
01d Med													9
01d Surg													6
: :													: :
: :													: :
: :													: :
15c Med													13
15c Surg													8
15e Med													58
15e Surg													74
Contacts													239
Elective													232
Preventive													9,808
Total													30,757
Supply	2,266	840	8,347	457	30	279	329	1,084	382	77	14,440	13,206	

Specialty Category

The number of eye care providers in each cell to be filled in by the linear programming algorithm.

NOTE: Need has been adjusted by subtracting out work done by non-ophthalmologist physicians (see Table 3.9).

disease and rehabilitative groupings, and one each for cosmetic contact lenses, refractive surgery, and preventive care. The rightmost column provides the FTE requirements produced by the need spreadsheet computations. The need and demand numbers have already been adjusted downward by subtracting out work performed by nonophthalmologist physicians.[10] The bottommost row shows the total supply of eye care providers by subspecialty area. There are 41,737 FTE providers to perform 30,757 FTEs of work.

Because supply exceeds need, we sought to allocate providers so that all row totals are met and no column totals are exceeded (i.e., all conditions are treated by available providers). The linear programming algorithm fills in the entries in the table according to a criterion that we specified.

To set up the mathematical formulation, we let

x_{rc} be a number associated with the (r,c)th cell (row r, column c),
N_{rc} be a number of eye care providers allocated to the (r,c)th cell.

The algorithm attempts to maximize:

$$\sum_{r,c} x_{rc} * N_{rc}, \tag{5.1}$$

subject to the constraints:

$$\sum_{c} N_{rc} = \text{row total},$$

$$\sum_{r} N_{rc} \leq \text{column total}.$$

The goal is to choose numbers x_{rc} in such a way that the maximization solution N_{rc} will be meaningful.

_____

[10] This adjustment used the percentages in Table 3.9 and amounts to about two percent of the total, which was reported as 31,419 in the previous chapter.

In general, the higher the value of x_{rc} is, the higher will be the number N_{rc} that the linear program wants to assign to the cell. Conversely, if $x_{rc} = 0$, the linear program will set $N_{rc} = 0$, because the product $x_{rc}*N_{rc}$ does not contribute to making the sum of products larger.

The following considerations were used in setting the values of x_{rc}:

1. DPA and TPA optometrists, by law, are not allowed to perform surgery or prescribe most systemic medications or treatment. As designated by "no" in Table 3.7, those diseases that optometrists cannot treat are identified by zeroes in their cells.

2. DPA optometrists get the highest priority in the initial model in order to establish a lower bound estimate of DPA excess. Because TPA optometrists and ophthalmologists can substitute for any functions of DPA optometrists, we know that any excess in the number of other providers can replace DPA optometry assignments, increasing the DPA excess. Therefore, we can get both upper and lower bounds on the need for DPA optometrists using this initial allocation strategy. Thus, we put 5s in the cells in which, by law, DPA optometrists are able to function. *This is a strategy to make this initial model the most flexible and illustrative; it is not an allocation based on quality, cost, or other judgments.*

3. For similar reasons, the TPA optometrists get the next highest priority: Put 4s in the cells in which, by law, they are able to function. Again, this provides a lower bound on any excess, and does not reflect quality, cost, or other judgments.

4. The next priority is to allocate ophthalmologist subspecialists to their surgical area of expertise, in recognition of the perceived role and value of subspecialty training and experience. This maximizes the use of subspecialists in areas where they are particularly well trained, which we assume is desirable from a public health standpoint. To do this, put 3s

in those cells of the interaction of subspecialists and
subspecialty conditions only.

5. We allocate general ophthalmologists next, because if
   subspecialists are restricted to their specialty area of
   training (Step 4), we want to know how many subspecialists will
   be used. Giving general ophthalmologists 2s in all entries
   accomplishes this, if we also give ophthalmologist
   subspecialists 1s outside their surgical area of expertise.

Note that our choice of 1s through 5s has hierarchical significance
only; the linear programming assignment depends only on the ordinal
ranking of these numbers. Using 1s through 5s, Table 5.2 completely
defines the input to the linear program.

Reconciliation Results

The linear programming algorithm allocates eye care providers to
each cell of the previous table. These allocations add up to adjusted
need across rows, and add up to less than (or equal to) the total
supply. Thus, eye care needs are met with an excess of providers. Next
we focus on describing this excess.

Table 5.3 describes the results of our model runs, by year and by
three types of model (optometry-first, ophthalmology-first, and primary-
care provider). The three models allocate priorities differently. In
the first two, either optometrists or ophthalmologists are allocated all
the care they can provide; any unmet need or demand that they cannot
fill is then given to the other type of provider. In the last model,
optometrists and general ophthalmologists are allocated all care first,
with residuals (if any) then going to subspecialist ophthalmologists.
Within this model, care is allocated to optometrists first to provide
maximum flexibility; again, no quality or cost of care judgments are
implied.

The total number of FTE eye care providers currently required,
according to our estimate of need, is 30,757. In contrast, we have
14,091 FTE ophthalmologists and 27,646 FTE optometrists available, for a
total surplus of 10,980 FTEs. The surplus is estimated to grow to

Table 5.2
Assignments of Multipliers for the Linear Programming Algorithm

Grouping	Specialty Category												Adjusted Need
	CAT	COR	GEN	GLAU	LV	NEUR	PLAS	RET	STR	UV	DPA	TPA	
01a Med	1	1	2	1	1	1	1	1	1	1	5	4	1,567
01a Surg	3	1	2	1	1	1	1	1	1	1	0	0	2,788
01b Med	1	1	2	1	1	1	1	1	1	1	0	4	1
01c Med	1	1	2	1	1	1	1	1	1	1	0	4	1,812
01c Surg	3	1	2	1	1	1	1	1	1	1	0	0	1,229
01d Med	1	1	2	1	1	1	1	1	1	1	5	4	9
01d Surg	3	1	2	1	1	1	1	1	3	1	0	0	6
⋯	⋅	⋅	⋅	⋅	⋅	⋅	⋅	⋅	⋅	⋅	⋅	⋅	⋯
⋯	⋅	⋅	⋅	⋅	⋅	⋅	⋅	⋅	⋅	⋅	⋅	⋅	⋯
⋯	⋅	⋅	⋅	⋅	⋅	⋅	⋅	⋅	⋅	⋅	⋅	⋅	⋯
15c Med	1	1	2	1	1	1	1	1	1	1	0	4	13
15c Surg	1	1	2	1	1	1	1	1	1	3	0	0	8
15e Med	1	1	2	1	1	1	1	1	1	1	5	4	58
15e Surg	1	1	2	1	1	1	1	1	1	1	0	0	74
Contacts	1	1	2	1	1	1	1	1	1	1	5	4	239
Elective	3	3	3	1	1	1	1	1	1	1	0	0	232
Preventive	1	1	2	1	1	1	1	1	1	1	5	4	9,808
Total													30,757
Supply	2,266	840	8,347	457	30	279	329	1,084	382	77	14,440	13,206	

NOTE: Need has been adjusted by subtracting out work done by non-ophthalmologist physicians (see Table 3.9).

Table 5.3
Summary Description of Supply, Requirements, and Excesses,
by Model, Type of Provider, and Year

FTE Supplier Type	Supply	Optometry-First		Ophthalmology-First		Primary-Care Provider	
		Required	Excess	Required	Excess	Required	Excess
Need							
Gen	8,347	3,261	5,086	8,347	0	7,800	547
Spec	5,744	4,539	1,205	5,744	0	0	5,744
Tot-Oph	14,091	7,800	6,291	14,091	0	7,800	6,291
Optom	27,646	22,957	4,689	16,666	10,980	22,957	4,689
Total	41,737	30,757	10,980	30,757	10,980	30,757	10,980
Demand							
Gen	8,347	743	7,604	8,347	0	4,233	4,114
Spec	5,744	3,490	2,254	5,744	0	0	5,744
Tot-Oph	14,091	4,233	9,858	14,091	0	4,233	9,858
Optom	27,646	17,921	9,725	8,063	19,583	17,921	9,725
Total	41,737	22,154	19,583	22,154	19,583	22,154	19,583
Need, Year 2000							
Gen	8,220	3,896	4,324	8,220	0	8,220	0
Spec	6,608	5,010	1,598	6,608	0	686	6,608
Tot-Oph	14,828	8,906	5,922	14,828	0	8,906	5,922
Optom	29,531	25,335	4,196	19,413	10,118	25,335	4,196
Total	44,359	34,241	10,118	34,241	10,118	34,241	10,118
Need, Year 2010							
Gen	8,371	4,717	3,654	8,371	0	8,371	0
Spec	7,603	5,332	2,271	7,603	0	1,678	7,603
Tot-Oph	15,974	10,049	5,925	15,974	0	10,049	5,925
Optom	33,492	27,480	6,012	21,555	11,937	27,480	6,012
Total	49,466	37,529	11,937	37,529	11,937	37,529	11,937

NOTE: Need and demand have been adjusted by subtracting out work done by non-ophthalmologist physicians.

19,583 FTEs if only demand is considered; 22,154 FTEs could provide the eye care services currently demanded.

The allocations clearly show that there are excess providers of eye care. Under the optometry-first model scenario (with surgical care priorities going to the subspecialty ophthalmologists as opposed to general ophthalmologists, as would be likely in a postulated optometric-first model of care), there are over 4,500 surplus FTE optometrists and over 6,000 surplus FTE ophthalmologists; the surplus is relative to the number of FTEs sufficient to satisfy the public health need for eye care services. On the demand side, there would be a surplus of nearly 10,000 FTE optometrists and nearly 10,000 FTE ophthalmologists under the optometry-first model.

Under the ophthalmologist-first model, in which ophthalmologists provide routine primary eye care, there would be no surplus of ophthalmologists in any specialty area for either need or demand requirements. For demand, however, this would mean that over 5,000 FTEs would be engaged in preventive eye care services. The effect on optometry under this structure would be *severe* because optometrists would be displaced in a 1:1 relationship. Thus, in considering the demand for eye care services, if ophthalmologists provided all the primary care demanded, 71 percent of all optometrists would be surplus, since 14,091 ophthalmologists filling 22,154 FTEs would leave about 8,000 FTEs for optometrists. When need is considered, 16,666 optometrists would be required, resulting in a remaining total surplus of about 11,000 optometrist FTEs.

The primary care provider model postulates that generalist ophthalmologists can perform any of a subspecialist's functions. In this model, need can be satisfied without using any subspecialist ophthalmologists. Excess general ophthalmologists are shown to be 547 FTEs for current need and 4,114 FTEs for current demand under a system of full utilization of optometric capabilities. The results reported here assign optometrists first, but the model is in reality indifferent to optometrists being displaced by ophthalmologists. This displacement would decrease their surplus while increasing that of optometrists.

Table 5.4 shows FTEs needed and demanded for the optometry-first model. For need, we see that a surplus of ophthalmologists would exist for most ophthalmic subspecialties (except for strabismus, cataract, and glaucoma). For demand, we see a surplus in ophthalmologists in every specialty.

Table 5.4
Assignments from Linear Programming, Optometry-First Structure

Type of Provider	Year						
	1994			2000		2010	
	FTE Supply	FTEs Needed	FTEs Demanded	FTE Supply	FTEs Needed	FTE Supply	FTEs Needed
Cataract	2,266	2,266	1,844	2,185	2,185	1,844	1,844
Cornea	840	195	250	1,122	211	1,539	225
General	8,347	3,261	743	8,220	3,896	8,371	4,717
Glaucoma	457	457	307	653	653	952	867
Low Vision	30	0	0	30	0	38	0
Neuro	279	34	14	261	37	227	42
Plastics	329	214	173	317	229	284	241
Retina	1,084	969	691	1,399	1,113	1,815	1,271
Strabismus	382	382	186	558	558	815	815
Uveitis	77	22	25	83	24	89	27
DPA	14,440	14,440	14,440	12,020	12,020	8,801	8,801
TPA	13,206	8,517	392	17,511	13,315	24,691	18,679
Total	41,737	30,757	22,154	44,359	34,241	49,466	37,529

NOTE: Need and demand have been adjusted by subtracting out work done by non-ophthalmologist physicians.

In summary, under a primary care ophthalmology-first model, to meet public health need there would be a requirement for every available FTE ophthalmologist as well as 16,666 FTE optometrists: 10,980 FTE optometrists would be in surplus. Under a primary care optometry-first structure, there would still be a surplus of 4,689 FTE optometrists, but there would also be a surplus of 6,291 ophthalmologists.

The effect of the surplus by type of provider varies tremendously and depends mostly on how primary eye care is structured. As Table 4.4 shows, preventive care visits constitute over half of the demand requirements and over one-quarter of the need requirements. If preventive care guidelines were revised to indicate that more frequent exams were appropriate, preventive care services would constitute an even larger portion of the eye care workforce requirements.

These results are in line with expectations based on earlier workforce efforts. GMENAC estimated that roughly 11,000 FTEs would be required in 1990. Our results not only extend four more years into the future but are affected particularly by the inclusion of preventive care services and our ability to include care requirements for more eye diseases/conditions than GMENAC.

On the other hand, the estimates of the 1978-1984 study by the AAO (Ruiz, 1984) are closer to the results of the present study, particularly if preventive care FTEs are excluded. A comparison of the two studies shows that the AAO study used very different input data. Numerous data elements differ significantly, such as the definition of clinical population, the time required to perform surgery, and the number of follow-up visits required each year. However, the efficiencies introduced over the past 15 years into health care generally, and eye care in particular, allow for far greater numbers of patients to be seen and treated today than ever before. Thus, the estimated overall number of FTEs required from the AAO study and this study differ by less than 25 percent for meeting the need for problem-oriented care.

The results are also consistent with anecdotal evidence from the eye care community. Today, there is a sense that not all eye care providers are working at capacity; there is a *perceived* excess supply relative to demand. Yet there is also the realization that many people who would benefit from care do not receive care. Our results suggest that there is indeed capacity within the health care community to deliver services to those with unmet need.

The projection of the supply-to-requirements reconciliation shows a similar surplus in the future. Table 5.4 shows the projections for the years 2000 and 2010 for need, which reveal large future surpluses of eye care providers. The extent of the surplus is 10,118 FTEs in the year 2000, growing slightly to 11,937 FTEs in the year 2010. As today, the use of an ophthalmology primary care model would mean that there would be no surplus of ophthalmologists. Also as today, even the optometry-first model carries with it a significant surplus of optometrists. Any reduction in the work year or the use of longer time to provide similar care would serve to reduce the FTE equivalence and thus the number of FTE optometrists available, thereby reducing the surplus. Further, to the extent optometrists provide services not addressed in this model, the FTEs available would also be reduced (as discussed further in Chapter Six).

ROBUSTNESS OF THE RESULTS

Accounting for Uncertainty

Even though our results appear to reflect the current environment, we were concerned that the specified judgments and data extrapolations, combined with inherent variation and uncertainty in the data elements themselves, may affect the stability of these findings. To create a range of estimates within which we would have a high degree of confidence, we utilized bootstrap techniques and other statistical randomization schemes. These techniques caused all those data elements that were derived from survey data or based upon judgment to vary. Except for the number of work hours per year and the preventive visit schedule, every other variable in the modeling was varied in repeated bootstrap and simulation runs to determine the stability of the FTEs-required estimates (both need and demand).

Repeated bootstrap runs showed that the extremes of the range of FTEs required for need fell within the range 28,500 to 33,500 FTEs, with a standard error of about 1,500. Likewise, the surplus ranges from about 8,500 to 13,500 FTEs, with a standard error of 1,500. Surplus FTE optometrists under the optometry-first model have a mean of about 6,000 and a standard error of 1,200; surplus FTE ophthalmologists have a mean of about 4,500 and a standard error of 900.

Thus, we felt comfortable with the model's projections of the number of FTEs required as well as the supply of FTEs. All the inferences drawn are stable across parameter variations. We take no position on the desirability of the optometric over ophthalmic primary care model or vice versa in this study. However, it is important to note the consequences of choosing the alternative models for the different forms of independent eye care providers.

Optometrist / Ophthalmologist Work-Time Ratios

Information from the survey of 2,007 ophthalmologists practicing in the United States was conducted to determine the amount of time required to treat patients medically and surgically for specific eye conditions. Because the American Optometric Association did not participate in the study, a parallel survey of optometrists was not conducted. Instead, a work-time ratio was used to reflect the potential differential amount of time optometrists require to provide eye care services compared to ophthalmologists for those conditions that optometrists are legally allowed to provide medical care. Because anecdotal evidence and optometric trade journals suggest that the number of hours worked each year by the average optometrist may be less than that of an average ophthalmologist, and that the amount of time used by optometrists in caring for patients may be longer, a range of work-time ratios between 0.6 and 1 was used and workforce estimates provided for each ratio. The work-time ratio of 1 reflects the null hypothesis that both types of providers supply the same amount of patient care time per year and use the same amount of time to care for patients. A work-time ratio of 0.6 reflects an alternative hypothesis that optometrists supply fewer patient care hours, provide services not covered in this study, and/or take more time in the care of patients. The work-time ratio does not imply differences or equivalencies in the quality or cost-effectiveness of care; it is an analytical device used to overcome the lack of data concerning optometric-specific work times. In addition, the work-time ratio is a way to incorporate the impact of optometric services that have not been included explicitly in this study.

Table 5.5 shows how the current demand and need for eye care providers vary as as the work-time ratios for optometrists decrease. Regardless of the type of health care delivery system, the estimated need and demand for services is constant because the same work times and FTE definitions are used. Thus, there is a current requirement of 30,757 FTE eye care providers to satisfy the population's need for services, and a requirement of 22,154 FTE eye care providers to satisfy the population's demand for services. The simple comparison of supply and demand or need shows that a surplus exists relative to demand across the range of work-time ratios for optometrists. This surplus is robust to the data, with a standard error of about 2,000 FTEs.

Table 5.5
Demand and Need for Eye Care Services Relative to Supply

Work-Time Ratios	Number of FTE Optometrists	Number of FTE Ophthalmologists	Total FTE Supply	FTEs Demanded	FTEs Needed
1.0	27,646	14,091	41,737	22,154	30,757
0.8	22,117	14,091	36,208	22,154	30,757
0.6	16,588	14,091	30,679	22,154	30,757

Table 5.6 presents the results of reconciliation when public health need is allocated to optometrist or ophthalmologist providers under the two extreme boundary scenarios: optometrists first and ophthalmologists first. As stated above, a range of estimates was calculated, reflecting different work-time ratios for optometrists. The results indicate that ophthalmologists would be in surplus only in the optometry-first model. Optometrists, on the other hand, are in surplus, except when the work-time ratio is 0.6 or less in the ophthalmologist-first model or when the work-time ratio is 0.8 or less in the optometry-first model. Again, these results highlight the need for additional data to better understand optometric care patterns and to determine the appropriate work-time ratio.

Table 5.6
Allocation of Care Under Two Delivery-System Scenarios,
Public Health Need

Type of Provider and Work-Time Ratios	Supply	Optometry-First		Ophthalmology-First	
		Required	Excess	Required	Excess
Ophthalmology	14,091	7,800	6,291	14,091	0
Optometry					
1.0	27,646	22,957	4,689	16,666	10,980
0.8	22,117	22,957	0	16,666	5,451
0.6	16,588	22,957	0	16,666	0

NOTE: Under a 0.6 work-time ratio for the optometrist-first model, the net effect is to eliminate the ophthalmologist surplus.

RAND Eye Care Workforce Survey: Response Bias Effects

The response rate to the survey was 40 percent. We performed two separate analyses to see if there was any response bias.

Early Response. The first analysis determined whether those who responded early differed from those who responded late (after two rounds of reminders). We partitioned the survey responses into three groups, which corresponded roughly to those who responded within the first ten days after receiving the survey, those who responded later but before a reminder notice was sent out, and those who responded after receiving a second packet and reminder notice. We pretended that each of these groups was the universe of responders, and we carried out three separate need and reconciliation estimations, in which the time estimates for care and the proportion undergoing surgery were based on each group. The resulting estimates of need and excess suppliers were within 1,500 of each other. Total need was 30,646, 32,113, and 31,809 for the early, middle, and late responders, with surpluses of 11,091, 9,624, and 9,928, respectively. These and other surpluses from the reconciliation model were consistent with the results described earlier. We concluded that timing of response would not affect our basic conclusions.

Survey Population Characteristics Versus Respondent Characteristics. The second analysis compared the demographic and practice characteristics of survey respondents with those of the general survey population (see Table 5.7). We judged that the responding and full populations compared quite well along most dimensions, the lone exception being age. Respondents tended to be younger than nonrespondents; on average, they were three years younger than the full AAO ophthalmologist population.

To investigate the possible biases due to age, we split the population in half and ran separate analyses on each half, deriving survey estimates of time and estimates of need, and carrying out a reconciliation. The results were interesting. The younger age group yielded medical work times that were about the same as the older group's, but their surgical times were 40 to 50 percent longer. The net effect was a higher need estimate of 32,588 FTEs based on the younger group's times, and lower 29,454 based on the older group's times, compared with the 30,757 reported in Table 5.3. We conclude that age response bias could have led to a slight overestimate of need (about 1,000 FTEs), adding further support to the basic findings of surplus.

Stability Across Census Regions

A concern for workforce studies is the geographic distribution of any surplus or shortage of providers. Indeed, even today, inner-city neighborhoods and poor rural areas often lack easily accessible health care. Unfortunately, localizing workforce allocations to specific counties or zip codes carries significant methodological risks because of factors that are important but difficult to incorporate, such as transportation, boundary-crossing to seek care, and time as opposed to distance considerations. Moreover, many providers have multiple offices, often located in different zip codes or counties, and it is impossible using current data sources to allocate these providers precisely. Further, any specific geographic unit is itself artificial: An area with a shortage of health care professionals may exist on paper for one side of a street but not for the other. For these and other reasons, such as the mobility of ophthalmologists and the presence of multiple satellite offices, we did not allocate the workforce

Table 5.7
Comparison of Full Survey Population with Responding Survey Population

Characteristic	Value	Full Sample	Respondent
U.S. Born	yes	87.8	90.4
Census Region	North	24.5	19.5
	Central	21.0	25.7
	South	32.6	30.6
	West	21.8	24.2
Board Certification	blank	9.6	5.2
	ABO	90.4	94.8
Practice Type	blank	18.5	16.8
	ADMIN	.0	.0
	CONSULT	.0	.0
	GROUP	29.9	28.9
	HMO	1.6	1.9
	HOSPITAL	.2	.3
	MILITARY	1.1	2.5
	MULTI	2.9	4.5
	RESEARCH	.0	.0
	RETIRED	5.4	.0
	SCIENTIST	.0	.0
	SOLO	35.3	29.6
	UNIVERSITY	4.8	15.6
	VOLUNTEER	.0	.0
AAO Status	FELLOW	88.1	91.7
	INTERNAT.	.6	.0
	TRAINING	11.3	8.3
Average Age		49.4	45.0

reconciliation to small geographic areas. Even preliminary estimates by states reflected these concerns. When better data become available on what would constitute a reasonably contained market, with boundaries, for eye care services, the model can be used to project workforce requirements for that region.

In the interim, we elected to use the four census regions to represent geographic distribution. Given the large surplus that exists, a region even approaching equilibrium would be a relatively more desirable location in which to establish a practice than one that showed a large surplus of providers.

As seen in Table 5.8, no region approaches equilibrium. Furthermore, the surplus appears to be evenly distributed across the four census regions, although the South appears to have the smallest surplus.

Table 5.8
Distribution of Reconciliation Across Census Regions

Region	Need	Supply
Midwest	7,468	10,265
North	6,474	9,065
South	10,584	11,890
West	6,232	10,518

SUMMARY

The reconciliation of the workforce models shows that there is a significant surplus of eye care providers. This conclusion is stable. How this surplus affects the different providers of eye care depends on the structure of the delivery system. Also, no census region of the country currently has a shortage of eye care providers, although the South has the smallest surplus. The next chapter discusses the implications of these findings and the conclusions drawn from the modeling.

6. CONCLUSIONS AND POLICY IMPLICATIONS

The reconciliation of the available supply of eye care providers and the requirements for such services, as defined by either public health need or demand/utilization (Chapter Four), shows that more FTE eye care providers are available than are required. This finding holds regardless of who (e.g., optometrist, ophthalmologist, or other physician) provides the eye care services. When only demand is examined, we find there is an even larger surplus of eye care providers. Further, the surplus of eye care providers continues through the year 2010, despite the aging of the U.S. population.

This chapter explores these central findings in greater detail. It examines the effects of the structural decisions and assumptions we used in our modeling on the conclusions, compares our findings with those of other workforce studies and methodologies, and considers the implications of our findings for potential workforce policy.

EXCESS RELATIVE TO DELIVERY SYSTEM

Our analyses show that there is a current excess supply of eye care providers of between 8,000 and 14,000 FTEs relative to public health need. How the excess supply is divided between ophthalmologists and optometrists depends on the structure of the eye care delivery system and whether demand or need is considered. We examined three scenarios: optometrists as the primary eye care providers, ophthalmologists as the primary eye care providers, and a primary-care provider model using optometrists and general ophthalmologists as the primary care providers.

Optometrists are in oversupply under all three scenarios, with the excess ranging from 4,689 FTEs in the primary care optometry model to nearly 11,000 FTEs in the primary ophthalmology care model. The primary-care provider model shows an excess of from 4,689 to 5,236 optometrists, depending on whether they are displaced by general ophthalmologists in this setting. This excess would increase to 7,502 FTEs if cataract "specialists" were considered general ophthalmologists.

In the extreme scenario where ophthalmologists provide the primary eye care services, only 16,666 optometric FTEs are needed.

The picture for ophthalmologists, on the other hand, is less clear-cut. There is no excess of ophthalmologists when they are primary eye care providers. But in a delivery system that uses optometrists as the primary eye care provider, there is a surplus of over 6,000--only 7,800 FTE ophthalmologists are needed for the operative and systemic medical care of patients.

Comprehensive Ophthalmology

When we examined the supply of ophthalmologists, we exploited the generalist/specialist distinction so that we could address the current interest in *comprehensive ophthalmology*: a primary-care provider model. The requirements for subspecialist ophthalmologists can vary from zero to all that are available according to how ophthalmic surgical care is assigned. When we consider the workforce requirements for public health need under an ophthalmologist-first scenario, there is no subspecialty surplus; all 5,744 subspecialty FTEs are required. However, under the comprehensive primary-care provider model, virtually no subspecialist ophthalmologists are required. Under the primary optometric care model, while subspecialists provided all the surgical care and were restricted to providing *only* surgical care, there is still an excess of subspecialists in most ophthalmic subspecialty areas. Only when a significant portion of the medical office care is included as a component of surgical treatment are all subspecialists allocated. *Clearly, a policy designed to enhance the skills of comprehensive ophthalmologists to approximate those of subspecialists would reduce the need for subspecialists.*

Thus, it is clear that we need to understand how ophthalmologists (generalists and subspecialists) and optometrists can coordinate the care of their patients, especially surgical patients. For example, the ophthalmologist and optometrist comanagement of post-operative care is currently limited to cataract surgery. Data do not exist that specifically address the extent of optometric comanagement of cataract surgery patients. Referring to Medicare billing data for "post-operative care only," we estimate that approximately 75,000 cases annually involve optometric comanagement (Powell, 1991). However, the net effect of this level of comanagement is to transfer fewer than 40 FTEs (75,000 cases times 60 minutes for post-operative care divided by 2,016 hours per FTE) from the surgical care provided by ophthalmologists to the medical care of optometrists. If 1 million cataract cases each year were completely managed by optometrists in the post-operative period, the number of ophthalmologists required would be reduced by approximately 480 FTEs. Thus, a significant number of ophthalmologists are still needed, even under an optometry-oriented delivery system with extensive cataract surgery comanagement.

Relative Quality of Care Provided

Another issue that our results raise is the relative quality of care provided by ophthalmologists (generalists and subspecialists) and optometrists. We examined the supply of eye care providers under models that approximate different systems of care in which certain provider types receive priority in the allocation of patients. Ideally, the allocation should be made to maximize the quality of care provided (and received). We encountered two situations where such data would be useful to our model. First is the allocation of surgical patients. The implied questions are: Do subspecialist ophthalmologists provide higher-quality surgical care than comprehensive ophthalmologists? Is there a quality differential for all types of surgery or for only certain procedures? Second, is there a quality difference between optometrists and ophthalmologists for the care that both provide? If so, is there a quality differential for all types of care, or are any differences limited to certain types of care or conditions? These are crucial questions and there are few data to support an analysis by level of quality provided. Moreover, there are no data on the cost-effectiveness of different provider types, which would also enhance a workforce analysis.

Demand and the Surplus

The surplus of eye care providers is even more marked when demand or current utilization is considered. The current demand for 8,786 FTEs for medical and surgical problem-oriented care today may appear low, but it is consistent with independent evidence. A *Medical Economics* survey of ophthalmologists noted that 49 percent thought they were practicing below their capacity (Clark, 1990). In addition, this level of demanded supply is consistent with projections of workforce needs using staff model HMO ratios of ophthalmologists to enrollees. With 250 million persons in the United States, and a ratio of 1 ophthalmologist to every 33,333 persons (i.e., 3 ophthalmologists per 100,000 persons) there is a demand for approximately 7,500 FTE ophthalmologists (Weiner, 1994).

Our model narrowly defines elective and preventive care services. Current eye care practice patterns most likely use preventive care visits and elective services at rates higher than those envisioned by the AAO Preferred Practice Patterns and National Eye Care Forum consensus recommendations. Indeed, a survey of ophthalmologists in *Ophthalmology Times* (July 1989, p. 30) noted that the greatest single reason for patient visits was for "routine" care. Further, the American Optometric Association estimated in 1993 that there were 78 million primary eye exams, 32 percent of which were delivered by ophthalmologists and 68 percent by optometrists (Bennett and Aron, 1993). These percentages would translate into 53 million primary care exams by optometrists and 25 million by ophthalmologists. Our model postulated the need for 50 million preventive care visits per year for the nation using the recommendations from the AAO Preferred Practice Patterns and the 1994 National Eye Care Forum Consensus Conference. In addition, the AOA and the Contact Lens Association of Ophthalmology estimate that there were 23 million users of contact lenses in the United States in 1993; our model estimated that nearly 20 million regular users needed almost 2 million visits in addition to their routine care visits for problems with their lenses.

Summary

Thus, our workforce model shows that there is an excess of eye care providers and that this excess persists under different eye care delivery system scenarios that allocate optometrists and ophthalmologists using different levels of priority for primary eye care services. Our models narrowly define demand (and need) for elective services and preventive services, at levels that are most likely below what is currently used. However, the level of "routine" visits in the model follows the care patterns recommended by the National Eye Care Forum.

STRUCTURAL DECISIONS AND ALTERNATIVE MODELS

Analysis of prior workforce efforts reveals that baseline assumptions and structural model decisions are determining factors in the output of such models and help account for the variation in results (Feil et al., 1993). In this study, three critical structural decisions carry significant output implications: the number of work hours per year per FTE; the degree to which optometrists and ophthalmologists are similar in providing problem-oriented care; and the preventive services package of visits recommended by the AAO Preferred Practice Patterns and the 1994 National Eye Care Forum. We can predict the influence of these parameters on the results of our model as well as that of alternative decisions.

Number of Work Hours per Year

The number of work hours per year used in this analysis is 2,016. This number was selected after examining our survey results, comparing the survey result with similar data provided by the American Medical Association survey of medical practice, and discussing it (and its implications) with our advisory board and members of the AAO. In our discussions, there were arguments for both increasing and decreasing the number. However, the AMA figure represented an estimate that the majority felt approximated reality, given the diversity of ophthalmic practice. Varying the number of work hours has a readily predictable effect: Decreasing the number would increase the number of FTE eye care providers required and reduce the surplus; increasing it would decrease the number of FTE eye care providers required and increase the surplus. To bring supply into balance with need would require a 26 percent decrease in the number of work hours per FTE per year. An additional 28 percent decrease would then be required to balance supply with demand.

We set the total hours available for optometrists and ophthalmologists to be the same. However, there is some evidence that optometrists have shorter work schedules than ophthalmologists. A survey of optometrists in Oregon revealed that the average work week was 38 hours and 48 weeks per year (1,824 hours per FTE per year) compared with the median that we used of 42 hours per week of direct patient care and 48 weeks per year for ophthalmologists (Bleything, 1994). These data suggest that ophthalmologists may work approximately 10 percent more hours than optometrists.

The differential between optometric and ophthalmic practice can also be looked at using visits (although our study does not use a visit-based approach). A survey of optometrists shows that the mean number of patient visits provided in a year was 2,927 in 1992 (Bennett and Aron, 1993); data from the AMA indicate that ophthalmologists provide a mean of 5,106 patient visits annually (111 visits per week * 46 weeks) (AMA, 1993c). However, no data are available that describe whether the patients or the content and nature of these visits were similar. Thus, we cannot adjust the visit figures to be comparable between optometrists and ophthalmologists. Yet, if this differential is real, the current supply of almost 28,000 FTE optometrists would be reduced to 16,000 (28,000 * 2,927/5,106) FTEs.

Provider-Type Differences

A more complex issue to address is our use of a time equivalence between optometrists and ophthalmologists, and between generalist and subspecialist ophthalmologists for those services that are provided by both types of providers. Because the AOA did not participate in this study, we were unable to conduct a survey of optometrists that was comparable to our ophthalmologist survey, and to our knowledge there are no reliable published data on the relative time spent in providing eye care for similar patients among optometrists, ophthalmologists, and other physician providers.

We were able to obtain some anecdotal evidence concerning the time differential between optometrists, generalist ophthalmologists, and subspecialist ophthalmologists for several types of office visits. For eye examinations of new patients, optometrists took 70 percent longer than generalist ophthalmologists; for established patients, optometrists took 14 percent longer. However, for office visits, optometrists took about five percent less time than ophthalmologists. Generalist and subspecialist ophthalmologists took the same amount of time for office visits, but generalists took 40 percent longer for post-operative visits. However, these data may not be for comparable patients or comparable visits, owing to the small numbers of diagnoses in common. Nevertheless, the data do suggest that there may be time differentials on both the optometrist/ophthalmologist and generalist/subspecialist dimensions. These issues need to be explored further.

Another facet of these provider-type differences comes from the Cataract PORT study (Luthra et al., 1994), which found that optometrists tend to order more pre-operative tests for cataract patients than do ophthalmologists. Thus, the time it takes to order and interpret the test results may increase the overall time optometrists spend with cataract patients. However, there were no data on the content and time for the other components of the pre-operative exam visit. Thus, more information is clearly needed to examine the case-mix and service provision of optometric and ophthalmic provider practices.

Preventive Services Package

The final parameter that we held constant concerns the preventive screening schedule for children that was developed at the 1994 National Eye Care Forum and the use of the AAO Preferred Practice Patterns (see Table 2.5). An alternative to this schedule is the American Optometric Association's preventive screening program, which includes annual visits up to age 18, visits every two years until age 60, and annual visits thereafter. Implementation of the AOA's recommendations would require 15,000 FTEs to provide preventive care services, which is 6,000 FTEs greater than the preventive visit need estimates used in this model.

It is possible to analytically decrease (or increase) the surplus of eye care providers by manipulating these three parameters. If we reduce the number of hours worked per year, of both optometrists and ophthalmologists, and adopt the AOA preventive screening schedule, we could eliminate the surplus of providers, both optometrists and ophthalmologists, and bring supply into equilibrium with public health need. *Decreasing the number of work hours per year, incorporating time differentials between optometrists and ophthalmologists (i.e., increase the optometric time required to care for a given patient type relative to the ophthalmologist time), and adopting the AOA schedule of preventive visits increases the FTEs required, thus, decreasing the surplus of eye care providers.*

Conceptual Framework

It is important to remember the conceptual framework for this study, which partitions eye care services into four domains of care: problem-oriented, rehabilitation, elective, and preventive services. This framework, however, may not capture other services that ophthalmologists or optometrists provide. For example, we have not included the resources required to provide vision therapy and eye muscle exercises. To the extent that such services are needed (or demanded) and require time beyond that allocated to the treatment of the disease, the provision of these services would increase the time required and reduce the optometric surplus. However, few data exist that would enable such services to be inventoried, a classification derived, and time resources and frequencies of occurrence to be quantified. Without the participation of the AOA, such data remain unavailable.

Health Care Structure and Financing: Work Hour Changes

Health care structure and financing changes may also exert influence on one of the key parameters we used in our study: the annual number of work hours per FTE. To the extent that health care reform reduces paperwork and administrative burdens and providers continue to work the same number of hours, more hours will be available to spend in patient care activities, increasing the number of patient care work hours per year and, thus, decreasing the number of FTEs required. Similarly, if reimbursement levels decline, providers may work longer hours in an attempt to maintain income; this too would increase the number of patient care work hours per year and decrease the number of FTEs required. In contrast, increasing administrative activities and other factors, such as more intrusive case-management requirements, may reduce the provider surplus by reducing the patient care work hours available per year (Schwartz et al., 1988).

Other Influences on Workforce Size

Two final issues concerning factors that may affect the size of the workforce are the use of other personnel and the introduction of new technology.

Use of Other Personnel. We addressed the requirements for ophthalmologists and optometrists, and assumed that the number of other physician providers would always be sufficient to care for that fraction of eye conditions that present to nonophthalmologist physicians. We did not address the use of allied providers, such as ophthalmic technicians and ophthalmic registered nurses, for a number of reasons. First, while we requested information in our ophthalmologists' survey, it became clear that we could not adequately quantify a surplus (or deficit) because there are other tasks such personnel perform that were not included in our survey. Thus, we are unable to account for the tasks that define their daily routine. Second, the amount of training required is considerably less than that of optometrists or ophthalmologists. Consequently, the lead time for increases or decreases in the labor market is shorter. We can, however, predict how allied professionals affect optometrist and ophthalmologist patient care time: *The use of allied professionals should increase the time available of optometrists and ophthalmologists for patient care. If extensive use of such personnel is made, the surplus of providers will be increased.*

New Technologies. The effect of new technologies on optometric and ophthalmic practice is harder to predict. To the extent that new procedures or pharmaceuticals render previously inoperable or untreatable conditions treatable, the number of FTEs required will also increase. To the extent that new technologies increase the efficiency of providers so that they are able to see and treat patients more quickly, the number of FTEs required will decrease. We asked subspecialty societies and others to identify new areas of care in this regard; there was no consensus other than that refractive surgery will increase. Thus, we did not include additional changes in our future projections of the potential effects of new technology.

Need and Surplus

Finally, the public health need estimates are based on the number of persons who have an eye condition that requires treatment; implicit is the understanding that the health care system permits access to care and that patients seek (and complete) that care. Such an ideal situation may never be attained. Thus, the surplus of eye care providers will be larger than that reported above, because the number of FTEs required to meet the needs of all persons with eye disease is greater than the number required to meet the need of persons who will seek or be able to obtain care.

COMPARISON TO OTHER WORKFORCE METHODOLOGIES

The results of our study are consistent with the conclusions of earlier workforce studies, such as GMENAC, which showed an excess of eye care providers. More recent studies, such as the *Third Report of the Council on Graduate Medical Education to Congress*, have examined the supply and demand for physicians, combining ophthalmologists with other surgical subspecialties. These studies have found an excess of surgical specialists, which include ophthalmologists. However, none of the recent studies considers the coexistence of different types of independent providers. With the passage of state legislation expanding the scope of the practice of optometrists, as well as federal legislation that includes optometrists in federal health programs, workforce planning needs to take into account the contributions of optometrists. Our results suggest that among eye care providers, there is a clear excess of optometrists and there is most likely an excess of ophthalmologists.

The rapid growth of managed care plans has increased the policy interest in medical workforce issues. Such plans also provide an alternative framework for considering workforce issues. Recent workforce studies use physician staff-to-enrollment ratios to extrapolate workforce estimates to the entire U.S. population. These studies indicate that surgical specialists may be in excess supply by 60 to 80 percent (Weiner, 1994; Schroeder, 1994; Wennberg et al., 1993; Kronick et al., 1993; Mulhausen and McGee, 1989). Translated into FTEs, managed care plans using staff model HMO patterns would need only 7,700 to 8,750 FTE ophthalmologists.

Although the findings of these studies are similar to ours qualitatively, their focus is on ophthalmologists as opposed to *all* eye care providers. Yet implicit in the use of HMO staffing ratios is that other supporting staff, including optometrists, are available for patient care. The HMO staffing ratios also implicitly incorporate the traditionally lower numbers of patients seen per physician. Thus, a real issue in the workforce policy debate is how the health care system will be structured so that staffing patterns can better meet public health need as well as current demand.

One report of HMO staffing patterns revealed that the ophthalmologist staffing ratios of seven plans averaged 2.9 FTE ophthalmologists per 100,000 population. This level of staffing is below the ophthalmologist-to-population ratio reported by the GMENAC as being "needed," that is, 4.8 ophthalmologists per 100,000 population (Mulhausen and McGee, 1989). One clear implication is that managed care plans may configure their staff to de-emphasize ophthalmologist providers.

We estimate that these plans would have to employ between 15,000 and 20,000 FTE optometrists to provide the remainder of the required care, even excluding the elective care component of the model, if they persist at current ophthalmologist staffing ratios. As noted above, however, HMO staffing patterns are consistent with meeting current levels of utilization or demand for problem-oriented care and preventive services only. They do not accommodate demand for services that may be outside the traditional set of benefits, such as refractive surgery. To be more explicit, *HMO staffing ratios do not reflect a system designed to deal with the public health need of the U.S. population.*

Finally, the HMO staffing ratios are generally derived from plans of employed populations, so that those 65 years of age and older are underrepresented. This is particularly significant since the elderly consume about 50 percent of eye care visits (as estimated from the

NAMCS). Thus, the HMO staffing patterns may be inadequate for senior-oriented managed care plans, even with statistical corrections that reflect a 40 percent level of utilization by the elderly.

In addition, the influence of Independent Practice Associations and other alternative forms of managed care are less certain. No data are available on the effects posed by contractual arrangements or the inclusion or exclusion of eye care providers within these arrangements. Further, information on how these plans use different providers is lacking. The value of these data is magnified by the fact that staff model HMOs may not be economically viable in rural or less densely populated areas, necessitating the use of alternative forms of health care delivery organizations (Kronick et al., 1993).

Clearly, additional work is needed to better understand the effect of such changes, particularly non-staff-model managed care plans, on the mix of provider supply and requirements for eye care.

POLICY IMPLICATIONS

The results of this study carry four important policy implications: *First, there are more eye care providers than are required to meet the current level of demand for eye disease care, vision rehabilitation, and preventive care.* This conclusion must be interpreted with an understanding of the structural decisions and assumptions that underlie the modeling. Changes in the model's assumptions may significantly alter the strength of the conclusions or the extent of the surplus. However, under no likely eye care delivery system scenario is there a significant shortage of eye care provider supply to meet the demand.

We have also looked at public health need, defined by using population-based incidence- and prevalence-of-disease estimates, clinical practice patterns as determined from our survey of ophthalmologists, and preventive service recommendations of the National Eye Care Forum and the AAO Preferred Practice Patterns. Equilibrium of provider supply with need can occur only with adoption of the more generous American Optometric Association schedule of preventive services, or if data were to show that optometrists provide problem-oriented care at roughly half (0.6) the level of an ophthalmologist, owing to longer times per patient, other time commitments, shorter work weeks, or other factors.

The preceding discussion reveals some possible strategies to bring supply into line with demand. Providers can expand their elective care efforts; reduce the number of work hours per year either directly or indirectly (e.g., by use of job-sharing or other methods); or change the care patterns of eye conditions, preventive services, or rehabilitation. Adoption of the AOA preventive services schedule would be an example of this last strategy.

Second, more data are needed so that the skills and capabilities of the different types of eye care providers, including the optometrist/ophthalmologist and generalist/subspecialist comparisons, can be better optimized. We were able to construct three different eye care system scenarios. Reality falls somewhere within the bounds of these estimates. However, more data are needed so that allocations among providers can be made on the basis of measured quality-of-care or costs. Such data would provide a mechanism to determine workforce requirements with an explicit goal, such as determining the number of eye care providers (optometrists, ophthalmologists, and ophthalmic subspecialists) that would maximize quality of care, minimize costs, or maximize quality per unit cost.

Third, it is critical to continuously improve and update our knowledge of clinical practice, both in terms of the time involved and the patterns of care. Given the critical importance of these estimates, additional methodologies such as time-motion studies or work diaries to confirm, expand, and eventually supplant or at least supplement our survey results would be of value. To better reflect ongoing geographic patterns of care, it is important to document the true location of providers and the associated patient capacity, given that many providers have multiple contractual arrangements and office locations. Such data are necessary before we can conduct an analysis on small-area supply and need for eye care services.

Fourth, health care workforce planning must look at the level of public health need as well as current utilization or staffing patterns. For eye care services, we estimated demand to be about 70 percent of the public health need for services. What this ratio is for other types of medical problems, we do not know. Although it may be unrealistic to expect that the national health care system should staff at levels to provide 100 percent of the needed care, workforce planning must be cautious so that restrictions in specialty care training will not lead to shortages in the future. Such caution is particularly important today as the health care system evolves and as health care reform encourages change. As with so much of the health care planning in this country, the need to be cautious and to anticipate potential consequences (usually viewed as anticipatable in retrospect) should limit dogma supporting fundamental changes in workforce without additional data.

Appendix A

METHODS USED TO GROUP DIAGNOSES AND PROCEDURES
CREATING THE 97 DISEASE GROUPS AND THE 15 DISEASE CATEGORIES

As presented in Chapter Two, we envision four domains of care of eye care services: problem-oriented, rehabilitative or low vision, preventive, and elective. Each of these four domains can be defined primarily through diagnosis codes (problem-oriented and rehabilitative) or procedure descriptions (preventive and elective). In order to be precise about resource use (and hence workforce requirements), we must further define the problem-oriented and rehabilitative domains.

In order to implement the conceptual framework for the study, it was necessary for us to develop methods to handle health information (medical and epidemiologic) coming from a variety of sources. The organizing principle for much of these data is the consistent coding of diagnoses and procedures. Two coding systems are extant in the majority of health data systems: the International Classification of Disease, Ninth Revision (ICD-9), is used for both diagnostic and procedure coding, primarily for medical record coding and utilization surveys; and the Physicians' Current Procedural Terminology, Fourth Version (CPT-4), is used for procedure coding, primarily for billing purposes. This technical appendix describes our efforts to facilitate use of the available information.

CREATION OF THE LIST OF DIAGNOSES

Generally, utilization and epidemiologic data are diagnosis oriented, and as such, use the ICD-9 coding system or some variant of it. For example, ICD-9 diagnosis codes can be up to five digits; however, when precision in diagnosis is not required or reliable, abbreviated three- or four-digit diagnosis codes may be used.

Our first step was to identify those diagnosis codes in the ICD-9 coding system which relate to eye diseases. We began with a review of the American Medical Association (AMA) coding publications, and extracted all eye codes and codes potentially used by ophthalmologists.

Second, we generated frequency distributions for those diagnosis codes on visit records from ophthalmologists' offices using the National Ambulatory Medical Care Survey (NAMCS). These visit records present information describing a particular visit in a particular physician's office. Consequently, our frequency distributions identified diagnosis codes from visits originating from an ophthalmologist's office which were eye related as well as those codes which were not within the defined "ophthalmic" diagnosis code ranges from the AMA publications. We reviewed all of these potential "ophthalmic" diagnosis codes, and made a decision for each as to whether the diagnosis code represented one that an ophthalmologist might use in the routine care of eye patients. To provide additional information for this determination, we generated the relative frequency of each ICD-9 diagnostic code used by an ophthalmologist versus other physicians. Thus, our initial list of ophthalmic codes included the following types of diagnoses:

(1) all obvious eye codes (e.g., cataract),

(2) conjunctivitis, diabetes, and removal of superficial foreign bodies which are treated commonly by ophthalmologists and other physicians, and

(3) all other diagnosis codes which were used at least 75 percent of the time by ophthalmologists versus other physicians.

These diagnosis codes were the basis for our ambulatory-visit ophthalmic diagnosis code list, which accounted for more than 99 percent of all diagnoses recorded in ophthalmologists' offices.

Third, we analyzed the National Hospital Discharge Survey (NHDS) for those eye-related diagnosis codes that may be common in the hospital setting but are not often used in the ambulatory setting. Based on the potential range of diagnoses, as derived from AMA publications and the NAMCS, we generated a frequency distribution of the primary diagnosis codes from representative hospital discharge records. The final diagnosis list of ophthalmic codes accounted for more than 99 percent of all eye-related hospitalizations.

We combined the eye-related diagnosis codes identified in NAMCS and NHDS to generate a common listing of diagnosis codes. The diagnosis code list was again reviewed to ensure that all eye-related codes had been included. In particular, we carefully reviewed the use of three-through five-digit families of diagnosis codes, and all pertinent family codes were added to the final diagnosis code list.

The final list of ICD-9 diagnostic codes included over 1,000 individual disease codes. Many of these codes identified similar disease entities. In order to develop an analytically manageable number of "diseases," we aggregated diagnosis codes into 97 "disease groupings" (see Table 3.4). We used the following criteria to guide our aggregation of specific diagnosis codes into disease groupings:

(1) diagnosis codes which were clinically similar were included in the same grouping,

(2) minimize the clinical and patient management characteristic differences among diagnoses included in a group, and maximize the differences between diagnosis groupings, and

(3) maintain the commonly accepted disease groupings or lumping of different disease entities that already exist.

We then reaggregated the 97 disease groupings to create 15 disease categories. These 15 disease categories correspond closely with well recognized subspecialty boundary areas. Within the 97 disease groupings and 15 disease categories, there is a unique one-to-one assignment of diagnosis codes; that is, each diagnosis code is unique to one grouping. Moreover, each disease grouping is unique to one disease category.

Finally, our disease grouping structure was reviewed by numerous bodies: comments from the AAO coding committees, as well as input from AAO staff, ophthalmologists, and optometrists were incorporated to better refine these aggregations and assignments.

CREATION OF LIST OF PROCEDURES AND SERVICES

We used a similar approach to identify all eye-related procedure codes in various datasets which use the CPT-4 and ICD-9 procedure coding systems. First, we reviewed AMA publications and identified the potential range of procedure codes. The NHDS was examined to identify the ICD-9 procedure codes, and Medicare Part B counts (provided by the

National Eye Institute) were examined to identify frequently used CPT-4 procedure codes. For each file, we generated frequency distributions for the procedure codes. All eye-related procedure codes were identified; we tried not to miss any procedure code that might have been used to represent an eye procedure.

Unlike the development of the disease groupings and categories, we wanted to assign each procedure code to the disease grouping or groupings in which it may be used for the care of patients. Thus, we recognized that we could not have a unique one-to-one mapping of procedures to diagnoses. Second, we observed that there are a multiplicity of procedure codes which identify slight variations on a particular procedure. These slight differences, while clinically important, were not necessary to maintain for our purposes, and we did not want to have to depend on the accuracy of procedure code reporting. Thus while a cluster may consist of different procedures with different worktimes, no data system (and perhaps no ophthalmologist) can report data which can identify statistically distinct time estimates for individual procedure codes. For these reasons, we decided to develop clusters of similar procedure codes which could be assigned to our disease groupings. We used the following criteria in creating the procedure clusters:

(1) maintain the commonly recognized clinical procedure categories. For example, phaco vs. ECCE, or full thickness procedures vs. trabeculectomies vs. angle surgeries,

(2) maximize the potential similarities and minimize the differences in the time required to perform the procedures, and

(3) consider the experience of the average patient and the requisite time involved in the performance of any particular procedure.

An example of a procedure cluster is the following: while a pars plana vitrectomy for vitreous hemorrhage in a pseudophakic eye is distinct from a pars plana vitrectomy for traction retinal detachment with epiretinal membrane stripping, the latter is included with a pars plana vitrectomy, lensectomy, endolaser, and air-fluid exchange.

One important concern specific to procedure and service codes is that two different coding systems exist--the ICD-9 and CPT-4 systems. We needed to be able to combine the procedure lists derived from data sources which use the two procedure coding systems; the Medicare Part B billing data use modified CPT-4 codes, and the NHDS data use ICD-9 codes. We contacted the AMA, the California Medical Association, and several peer-review and commercial coding organizations to see if a "cross-walk" between these two coding systems was available. From these discussions, we concluded that no complete cross-walk linking equivalent ICD-9 and CPT-4 procedure codes existed. The California Medical Review Insititute did have a partial cross-walk. In addition, we did a complete review of the descriptors of each code, and built a cross-walk which included CPT-4 codes that map into multiple ICD-9 codes and vice versa. All such matches were analyzed and made internally consistent among codes. In addition, the system was reviewed to ensure that the multiply mapped codes were also consistent among the 97 disease groupings, so that the same CPT to ICD relationships were maintained for procedures across all 97 groupings.

LINKAGE OF DISEASES AND PROCEDURES AND SERVICES

We assigned each procedure cluster to a disease group or groups since one procedure may be used to treat multiple diseases. For example, trabeculectomy can be used for patients with primary open-angle glaucoma as well as secondary glaucoma. The procedure cluster which includes trabeculectomy is thus assigned to all glaucoma disease groupings.

Since no data are available on the time required to perform the variety of ophthalmic procedures, we conducted a survey of ophthalmologists to obtain disease- and procedure-specific worktimes. For the survey, we used disease groupings and procedure clusters as the surveyed units of observation. This was done to avoid surveying diseases (or procedures) which have little clinical distinction with regard to the resources required for treatment.

SUMMARY

We reviewed various data sources that provided health-related information and determined that these data were organized by diagnosis and procedure codes. Diagnoses were coded using the ICD-9 coding system, and procedures were coded using the ICD-9 and CPT-4 coding systems. Within each of these systems, there were too many eye-related codes to manage analytically. Thus, we developed 97 disease groupings, which aggregated to 15 disease categories, with the unique assignment of ICD-9 diagnosis codes to disease groupings (and categories). For procedures, we not only had to develop clusters of similar procedures, but we had to additionally develop a cross-walk between the ICD-9 and CPT-4 procedure coding systems. Our task of developing the procedure code cross-walk was made easier because of our use of procedure clusters. Thus, we were able to more accurately link like procedure codes from the two systems. We then assigned procedure clusters to disease group(s) according to current clinical practice patterns.

Our approach to the development of the disease groupings and the procedure clusters provides flexibility. When data providing more clinical detail are available, the methods used to develop more analytically manageable categories can be updated.

Appendix B
WORK TIME AND REQUIREMENTS ESTIMATES

Chapter Five presented parts of certain tables of summary information that were related to our spreadsheet calculations. The full tables contained entries for each of the 97 disease groupings, which we felt were too long to put in the text because they were simply reference material. This appendix reproduces those tables in their entirety. Tables B.1 and B.2 are counterparts to Tables 5.1 and 5.2, which provide worktime information and which are inputs to the spreadsheet computations. Table B.3 contains estimates of need and demand, which are outputs from the spreadsheet computations.

Table B.1
Components of Office Work Time

Disease Group and Description	Office Time			Percent Proceeding to Surgery	
	Initial Visit	Follow-up Visits		Laser	Incis
	Time	Freq	Time		
01a cataract	20	2	15	0	30
01b lens-related diseases	20	2	15	0	9
01c aphakia / pseudophakia	20	1	15	13	1
01d congenital cataract	30	2	15	4	12
02a severe conjunctivitis	13	2	10	0	0
02b conjunctivitis	10	1	10	0	0
02c conjunctival hemorrhage	10	1	10	0	0
03a corneal infection	20	6	15	0	7
03b immune keratitis	20	6	15	0	7
03c corneal edema	20	3	15	0	32
03d corneal dystrophy	20	2	15	1	13
03e corneal opacity	20	2	15	2	16
03f corneal deposits	20	2	11	2	10
04a blepharitis	10	2	10	0	0
04b dry eye	15	2	10	0	1
04c chalazion	14	2	10	0	38
04d pterygium	15	2	14	0	28
04e eyelid dermatitis	15	2	10	0	3
04f trichiasis	11	3	10	0	11
04g corneal / conjunctival mass	15	2	14	1	28
05a open-angle glaucoma	20	4	15	12	5
05b glaucoma suspect	25	2	15	3	0
05c narrow angle glaucoma	30	3	15	53	14
05d secondary glaucoma	30	4	15	10	15
05e congenital glaucoma	30	4	15	1	51
06a blindness	30	1	20	0	0
06b color blindness	30	1	20	0	0
06c one-eyed	30	1	20	0	0
06d visual impairment	30	1	20	0	0
07a optic neuropathy	40	4	20	0	4
07b visual disturbance (symptom)	40	2	20	0	0
07c visual field defect	36	3	20	0	0
07d cranial nerve abnormality	40	4	20	0	6

Note: Table continued on next page.

Table B.1
Components of Office Work Time (continued)

Disease Group and Description	Office Time			Percent Proceeding to Surgery	
	Initial Visit Time	Follow-up Visits		Laser	Incis
		Freq	Time		
07e other cns diseases	40	2	20	0	4
07f pupil abnormality	30	1	20	0	1
07g optic nerve abnormality	40	4	20	0	4
07h nystagmus	38	1	14	0	2
08a eyelid tumor	20	3	10	0	73
08b orbital inflammation	30	4	20	0	15
08c lacrimal gland disease	30	4	15	0	43
08d orbital mass	35	4	20	0	48
08e orbital deformity	30	4	15	0	44
09a external burns	20	4	10	0	19
09b stenosis NL system	20	2	10	1	51
09c ptosis	20	2	10	0	38
09d dacrocystitis	20	3	10	0	54
09e ectropion	20	3	10	0	63
09f entropion	20	3	10	0	72
09g external anomalies	20	2	15	0	19
09h tear duct abnormality	20	2	10	0	45
09i conjunctival scarring	20	4	10	0	19
09j other lid disease	20	2	15	0	19
10a myopia	15	1	15	0	0
10b refractive error	20	1	15	0	0
10c astigmatism	15	1	15	0	2
11a macular degeneration	20	2	15	4	0
11b diabetes	20	2	15	18	3
11c retinal detachment	30	3	15	9	90
11d vitreous opacities	20	2	20	0	8
11e retinal degeneration	28	1	20	3	0
11f arterial occlusion	28	4	15	27	3
11g macular pucker	30	2	15	0	22
11h crvo / brvo	28	4	15	28	3
11i chorioretinitis	30	4	20	2	3
11j vitreous deposit	20	2	20	0	8

Note: Table continued on next page.

Table B.1
Components of Office Work Time (continued)

Disease Group and Description	Office Time			Percent Proceeding to Surgery	
	Initial Visit	Follow-up Visits			
	Time	Freq	Time	Laser	Incis
11k retinal tumor	20	3	15	10	22
11l choroidal tumor	30	2	20	3	15
11m macular edema	25	4	15	27	3
11n macular cyst / hole	30	3	15	2	24
11o retinal vascular disease	25	2	15	20	4
11p RPE disorder	25	2	15	4	1
11q endophthalmitis	30	5	15	0	61
11r retinopathy of prematurity	25	3	15	5	3
11s intraocular anomalies	28	2	15	1	12
11t exudative / retinopathy	25	2	15	20	4
11u hiv	30	4	20	2	11
12a esotropia	20	3	15	0	34
12b exotropia	20	3	15	0	41
12c strabismus	30	2	20	0	17
12d vertical strabismus	27	3	15	0	49
12e amblyopia	20	4	15	0	4
13a superficial trauma	15	1	10	0	0
13b superficial foreign body	15	1	10	0	6
13c trauma (deep) foreign body	30	2	15	0	75
13d trauma (deep) orbital	30	2	15	0	57
13e sequelae trauma	28	4	15	0	48
13f ruptured globe	30	5	20	0	100
13g vitreous hemorrhage	30	4	20	29	22
13h hypotony	28	4	15	0	48
14a iridocyclitis	20	4	10	1	3
14b posterior uveitis	40	8	20	10	11
14c scleritis	35	6	15	0	3
15a herpes simplex	25	5	15	2	7
15b herpes zoster	30	4	15	4	11
15c iris lesions	30	2	20	3	15
15d other ocular infections	30	5	15	0	61
15e other	20	2	15	1	21

Table B.2
Components of Incisional and Laser Surgical Times

Disease Group and Description	Incisional Surgical Times (minutes)					Laser Surgical Times (minutes)				
	Pre-op	Intra-op	Same day	90-day Post-op		Pre-op	Intra-op	Same day	90-day Post-op	
				Freq	Time				Freq	Time
01a cataract	30	40	20	5	12					
01b lens-related disease	30	40	20	5	10					
01c aphakia / pseudo-phakia	30	35	15	4	10	20	10	5	2	10
01d congenital cataract	30	45	20	5	15					
02a severe conjunctiv-itis	12	10	0	1	10					
02b conjunctiv-itis	12	10	0	1	10					
03a corneal infection	30	30	15	5	10	20	10	5	2	10
03b immune keratitis	30	15	10	3	10	20	10	5	2	10
03c corneal edema	45	60	20	7	15					
03d corneal dystrophy	30	45	15	5	10	20	10	5	2	10
03e corneal opacity	45	60	15	6	10	20	10	5	2	10
03f corneal deposits	30	15	10	3	10	20	10	5	2	10
04a blepharitis	20	60	10	3	10					
04b dry eye	20	20	10	2	10					
04c chalazion	10	15	5	1	10					
04d pterygium	30	30	15	4	10					
04e eyelid dermatitis	20	60	10	3	10					
04f trichiasis	10	5	0	1	10					

Note: Table continued on next page.

Table B.2
Components of Incisional and Laser Surgical Times (continued)

Disease Group and Description	Incisional Surgical Times (minutes)					Laser Surgical Times (minutes)				
	Pre-op	Intra-op	Same day	90-day Post-op		Pre-op	Intra-op	Same day	90-day Post-op	
				Freq	Time				Freq	Time
04g corneal / conjunctival mass	30	35	15	4	10	20	10	5	2	10
05a open-angle glaucoma	45	60	20	10	12	30	15	10	4	10
05b glaucoma suspect	45	60	20	9	12	30	15	10	4	10
05c narrow angle glaucoma	30	30	15	6	10	30	20	12	4	10
05d secondary glaucoma	45	60	20	10	12	30	15	10	4	10
05e congenital glaucoma	45	60	20	8	14	30	20	12	4	10
06a blindness	40	75	20	4	10					
06c one-eyed	40	75	20	4	10					
06d visual impairment	40	75	20	4	10					
07a optic neuropathy	60	108	20	4	15					
07d cranial nerve abnormality	30	30	15	3	10					
07e other cns diseases	25	20	10	3	10					
07f pupil abnormality	30	15	10	3	10					
07g optic nerve abnormality	60	108	20	4	15					
07h nystagmus	60	108	20	4	15					
08a eyelid tumor	30	45	20	3	10					

Note: Table continued on next page.

Table B.2
Components of Incisional and Laser Surgical Times (continued)

Disease Group and Description	Incisional Surgical Times (minutes)					Laser Surgical Times (minutes)				
	Pre-op	Intra-op	Same day	90-day Post-op		Pre-op	Intra-op	Same day	90-day Post-op	
				Freq	Time				Freq	Time
08b orbital inflammation	40	75	20	4	14					
08c lacrimal gland disease	30	60	20	4	10					
08d orbital mass	40	60	20	4	10					
08e orbital deformity	35	60	20	3	10					
09a external burns	25	30	15	3	10					
09b stenosis NL system	20	15	15	2	10	20	10	5	2	10
09c ptosis	20	60	10	3	10					
09d dacrocystitis	25	45	15	3	10					
09e ectropion	20	60	10	3	10					
09f entropion	20	60	10	3	10					
09g external anomalies	35	60	20	3	10	20	10	5	2	10
09h tear duct abnormality	20	30	15	3	10					
09i conjunctival scarring	30	60	18	4	10					
09j other lid disease	30	60	18	4	10					
10a myopia	45	15	10	4	10					
10b refractive error	45	15	10	4	10					
10c astigmatism	45	15	10	4	10					
11a macular degeneration	35	70	15	5	15	30	20	10	2	15

Note: Table continued on next page.

Table B.2
Components of Incisional and Laser Surgical Times (continued)

Disease Group and Description	Incisional Surgical Times (minutes)					Laser Surgical Times (minutes)				
	Pre-op	Intra-op	Same day	90-day Post-op		Pre-op	Intra-op	Same day	90-day Post-op	
				Freq	Time				Freq	Time
11b diabetes	40	90	15	5	15	30	20	10	2	15
11c retinal detachment	40	60	15	4	15	30	20	10	3	15
11d vitreous opacities	38	60	19	5	15					
11e retinal degeneration	30	20	10	3	15	30	20	10	3	15
11f arterial occlusion	35	70	15	5	15	30	20	10	3	15
11g macular pucker	35	70	15	5	15					
11h crvo / brvo	35	70	15	5	15	30	20	10	2	15
11i chorio-retinitis	35	72	15	5	15	30	20	10	3	15
11j vitreous deposit	38	60	19	5	15					
11k retinal tumor	40	90	15	5	15	30	20	10	3	15
11l choroidal tumor	40	90	15	5	15	30	20	10	3	15
11m macular edema	35	70	15	5	15	30	20	10	2	15
11n macular cyst / hole	35	70	15	5	15	30	20	10	2	15
11o retinal vascular disease	35	70	15	5	15	30	20	10	3	15
11p RPE disorder	35	70	15	5	15	30	20	10	3	15
11q endophthal-mitis	30	45	15	5	15					
11r retino-pathy of prematurity	40	90	15	5	15	30	20	10	2	15

Note: Table continued on next page.

Table B.2
Components of Incisional and Laser Surgical Times (continued)

Disease Group and Description	Incisional Surgical Times (minutes)					Laser Surgical Times (minutes)				
	Pre-op	Intra-op	Same day	90-day Post-op		Pre-op	Intra-op	Same day	90-day Post-op	
				Freq	Time				Freq	Time
11s intra-ocular anomalies	40	70	15	4	15	30	20	10	3	15
11t exu-dative / retinopathy	30	20	10	3	15	30	20	10	3	15
11u hiv	30	20	10	3	15	30	20	10	3	15
12a esotropia	30	30	15	3	10					
12b exotropia	30	30	15	3	10					
12c strabismus	30	30	15	3	10					
12d vertical strabismus	30	30	15	3	10					
12e amblyopia	30	30	15	3	10					
13a superficial trauma	10	5	3	1	10					
13b superficial foreign body	10	5	3	1	10					
13c trauma (deep) foreign body	40	60	20	6	15					
13d trauma (deep) orbital	40	60	20	6	15					
13e sequelae trauma	40	60	20	6	15					
13f ruptured globe	40	60	20	6	15					
13g vitreous hemorrhage	30	45	15	5	15	30	20	10	2	15
13h hypotony	45	60	20	10	12	30	15	10	4	10
14a irido-cyclitis	30	15	10	3	10	30	30	12	3	15

Note: Table continued on next page.

Table B.2
Components of Incisional and Laser Surgical Times (continued)

Disease Group and Description	Incisional Surgical Times (minutes)					Laser Surgical Times (minutes)				
	Pre-op	Intra-op	Same day	90-day Post-op		Pre-op	Intra-op	Same day	90-day Post-op	
				Freq	Time				Freq	Time
14b posterior uveitis	38	82	20	4	15	30	30	12	3	15
14c scleritis	60	0	0	4	15	30	20	10	3	15
15a herpes simplex	30	20	10	4	10	30	30	12	3	15
15b herpes zoster	30	20	10	4	10	30	20	10	3	15
15c iris lesions	45	60	20	10	12	30	15	10	4	10
15d other ocular infection	30	45	15	5	15	30	20	10	3	15
15e other	30	40	20	5	12					

Table B.3
Final Estimates of Demand and Need from Spreadsheet

Condition	Need Med	Need Surg	Demand Med	Demand Surg	Need (2000) Med	Need (2000) Surg	Need (2010) Med	Need (2010) Surg
01a	1,567	2,788	904	1,541	1,836	3,266	2,124	3,781
01b	1	0	1	0	1	0	1	0
01c	1,812	1,229	467	303	2,122	1,438	2,460	1,668
01d	9	6	3	2	9	6	9	6
02a	14	0	14	0	15	0	15	0
02b	366	0	418	0	389	0	409	0
02c	17	0	18	0	19	0	20	0
03a	85	13	131	18	92	14	97	15
03b	0	0	0	0	1	0	1	0
03c	7	18	22	54	9	22	10	25
03d	52	37	54	39	56	40	59	42
03e	19	24	19	24	21	25	22	27
03f	0	0	0	0	0	0	0	0
04a	67	0	68	0	72	0	75	0
04b	49	2	55	2	53	2	56	2
04c	107	75	112	78	115	81	121	85
04d	36	46	36	46	38	49	40	52
04e	6	1	22	4	6	1	7	1
04f	7	1	7	1	8	1	8	1
04g	0	0	7	8	0	0	0	0
05a	1,115	410	654	243	1,324	487	1,540	565
05b	455	53	115	12	507	59	524	61
05c	87	149	22	39	102	173	110	188
05d	29	18	20	13	34	21	39	24
05e	6	25	0	1	7	27	7	29
06a	83	0	6	0	100	0	115	0
06b	2	0	3	0	2	0	2	0
06c	0	0	2	0	0	0	0	0
06d	519	0	0	0	615	0	725	0
07a	137	19	60	8	156	22	185	26
07b	89	0	143	0	97	0	106	0
07c	26	0	23	0	28	0	31	0
07d	43	5	59	6	46	5	49	5
07e	21	1	83	6	22	1	24	2
07f	16	0	2	0	17	0	19	0
07g	8	2	6	1	8	2	9	2
07h	13	2	0	0	14	2	15	2
08a	26	84	33	105	28	90	30	95
08b	22	11	80	38	24	11	25	12
08c	8	9	8	9	9	9	9	10

Note: Table continued on next page.

Table B.3
Final Estimates of Demand and Need from Spreadsheet (continued)

Condition	Need		Demand		Need (2000)		Need (2010)	
	Med	Surg	Med	Surg	Med	Surg	Med	Surg
08d	4	4	4	4	4	4	4	4
08e	0	1	0	1	0	1	0	1
09a	39	19	21	10	42	20	44	21
09b	42	59	42	59	45	64	47	67
09c	39	81	42	88	42	87	44	92
09d	11	22	11	22	12	24	12	25
09e	8	24	8	24	9	26	10	27
09f	8	22	8	22	8	23	9	25
09g	1	1	1	1	1	1	1	1
09h	5	10	5	10	5	10	5	11
09i	0	0	1	2	0	0	0	0
09j	3	2	9	9	3	3	3	3
10a	1,601	0	313	0	1,725	0	1,812	0
10b	2,107	0	549	0	2,271	0	2,383	0
10c	180	31	42	6	194	34	204	35
11a	788	122	115	17	936	145	1,109	171
11b	422	599	76	107	486	690	558	793
11c	7	27	75	297	8	30	9	32
11d	22	10	117	55	25	12	29	14
11e	7	1	10	2	9	2	10	2
11f	16	12	24	19	18	14	21	16
11g	6	11	9	14	7	13	9	14
11h	22	15	23	16	25	17	29	20
11i	3	0	14	2	3	0	3	0
11j	0	0	1	1	0	0	1	1
11k	1	1	1	1	1	1	1	1
11l	1	1	5	5	1	1	1	1
11m	30	18	27	16	35	21	40	24
11n	19	23	23	28	22	27	25	31
11o	28	31	25	25	33	35	38	41
11p	15	3	8	2	16	4	17	4
11q	6	9	20	33	7	11	8	13
11r	29	7	5	1	29	7	28	7
11s	61	53	8	6	65	56	68	59
11t	3	2	1	1	3	3	4	3
11u	5	1	2	0	5	1	5	1
12a	245	233	44	43	259	247	270	257
12b	321	433	23	33	352	473	377	508
12c	20	10	40	20	19	10	19	10
12d	85	138	8	12	93	151	106	172

Note: Table continued on next page.

Table B.3
Final Estimates of Demand and Need from Spreadsheet (continued)

Condition	Need Med	Need Surg	Demand Med	Demand Surg	Need (2000) Med	Need (2000) Surg	Need (2010) Med	Need (2010) Surg
12e	290	28	46	5	312	30	329	32
13a	17	0	109	0	17	0	17	0
13b	31	3	92	9	31	3	30	3
13c	40	155	1	6	42	164	43	168
13d	3	9	7	25	4	9	3	9
13e	0	1	2	4	0	1	0	1
13f	7	18	10	25	7	18	7	18
13g	4	5	17	19	4	5	4	5
13h	0	0	1	1	0	0	0	0
14a	98	10	98	10	106	11	111	12
14b	5	1	0	0	5	1	5	1
14c	55	3	55	3	59	3	62	3
15a	3	0	3	0	3	0	3	0
15b	1	0	15	4	2	0	2	1
15c	13	8	9	6	13	9	14	10
15d	0	0	1	2	0	0	0	0
15e	58	74	30	37	62	79	65	84
Contact lens	239	0	239	0	257	0	270	0
Refractive surgery	0	232	0	232	0	250	0	263
Preventive	9,808	0	12,897	0	10,498	0	11,004	0
Total	23,808	7,611	19,069	4,003	26,242	8,705	28,430	9,843

REFERENCES

American Academy of Ophthalmology, *Insights Into Primary Eye Care*, San Francisco, California: AAO, 1989.

American Academy of Ophthalmology, *National Eye Care Forum Preventive Eye Care Services Schedule*, San Francisco, California: AAO, 1994.

American Medical Association, *Physicians' Current Procedural Terminology (CPT-94)*, Department of Physician Data Services, Division of Survey and Data Resources, Chicago, Illinois: AMA, 1993a.

American Medical Association, *Physician Characteristics and Distribution in the United States*, Department of Physician Data Services, Division of Survey and Data Resources, Chicago, Illinois: AMA, 1993b.

American Medical Association, *Physician Marketplace Statistics*, Department of Physician Data Services, Division of Survey and Data Resources, Chicago, Illinois: AMA, 1993c.

American Optometric Association, *Caring for the Eyes of America: A Profile of the Optometric Professions, 1992*, St. Louis, Missouri: AOA, 1993.

Association of Schools and Colleges of Optometry (ASCO), *Annual Survey of Optometric Educational Institutions*, Rockville, Maryland, 1993.

Association of University Professors of Ophthalmology, *Ophthalmology Match Report--January 1993*, San Francisco, California, 1993.

Bennett, I., and F. Aron, "State of the Profession: 1993," *Optometric Economics*, Vol. 64, No. 10, October 1993, pp. 8-13.

Bleything, W. B., "A Profile of Optometric Practice," *Optometric Economics*, March 1994, pp. 32-34.

Blue Book of Optometry, *1993--1994 Who's Who in Optometry*, Butterworth-Heineman, Newton, MA, 1993.

Bureau of Health Professions, *Area Resource File*, Prepared by the Office of Data Analysis and Management, Rockville, Maryland: BHPr, September 1992.

Clark, L., "Are You Seeing Your Fair Share of Patients?" *Medical Economics*, Vol. 67, No. 24, December 1990, pp. 85-95.

Duke-Elder, S., *System of Opthalmology, Vol. 3, Normal and Abnormal Development*, St. Louis, Mo.: Mosby, 1964.

Efron, B., and R. J. Tibshirani, *An Introduction to the Bootstrap*, Chapman and Hall, Inc., New York, 1993.

Feil, E. C., H. G. Welch, and E. S. Fisher, "Why Estimates of Physician Supply and Requirements Disagree," *JAMA*, Vol. 269, No. 20, 1993, pp. 2659-63.

Flexner, A., *Medical Education in the United States and Canada*, Carnegie Foundation for the Advancement of Teaching, New York, 1910.

Gamble, L., A. J. Mash, T. Burdan, R. S. Ruiz, and B. E. Spivey, "Ophthalmology (Eye Physician and Surgeon) Manpower Studies for the United States: Part IV Ophthalmology Manpower Distribution 1983," *Ophthalmology*, Vol. 90, No. 8, 1983, pp. 47A-64A.

Graduate Medical Education National Advisory Committee (GMENAC), *Report of the Graduate Medical Education National Advisory Committee to the Secretary, Department of Health and Human Services: Vols. I--VII*, Washington, DC: Department of Health and Human Services Publ. No. (HRA) 81-651-657, 1981.

Greenberg, L., *Forecasting the Future Supply of Physicians: Logic and Operation of the BHPr Physician Supply Model*, Washington, DC: Department of Health and Human Services Publ. No. (OHPAR) 3-93, November 1992.

Greenfield, S., E. C. Nelson, M. Zubkoff, W. Manning, W. Rogers, R. L. Kravitz, A. Keller, A. R. Tarlov, and J. E. Ware, "Variations in Resource Utilization Among Medical Specialties and Systems of Care," *JAMA*, Vol. 267, No. 12, 1992, pp. 1624-1630,

Hsiao, W. C., L. Rand, D. K. Verilli, E. R. Becker, P. Braun, D. L. Dunn, J. Dernberg, and D. B. Yntema, *A National Study of a Resource-Based Relative Value Scale for Ophthalmology Services: Phase II, Final Report*, submitted to the American Academy of Ophthalmology, 1991.

International Classification of Diseases, Ninth Revision (ICD-9), DHHS Publication Number 91--1260, Health Care Finance Administration, U.S. Department of Health and Human Services, October 1991.

Kindig, D. A., J. M. Cultice, and F. Mullan, "The Elusive Generalist Physician: Can We Reach a 50% Goal?" *JAMA*, Vol. 270, No. 9, 1993, pp. 1069--1073.

Kriesberg, H. M., J. Wu, E. D. Hollander, and J. Bow, *Methodological Approaches for Determining Health Manpower Supply and Requirements, Volume I: Analytical Perspective*, Washington DC: DHEW Publication HRA 76/14511, 1976a.

Kriesberg, H. M., J. Wu, E. D. Hollander, and J. Bow, *Methodological Approaches for Determining Health Manpower Supply and Requirements.*

Volume II: Practical Planning Manual, Washington DC: DHEW Publication HRA 76/14512, 1976b.

Kronick, R., D. C. Goodman, J. Wennberg, and E. Wagner, "The Marketplace in Health Care Reform: The Demographic Limitations of Managed Care," *NEJM*, Vol. 328, No. 2, 1993, pp. 148-152.

Lewin-VHI, *Base year Physician Utilization by Specialty, Activity, and Patient Demographics*, Contract 240-90-0067, May 1992.

Luthra, R., E. B. Bass, et al., "Optometrists' Use of Pre-Operative Testing in Cataract Patients," *Investigative Ophthalmology and Visual Science*, Vol. 34, 1994, p. 1225.

Mulhausen, R., and J. McGee, "Physician Need: An Alternative Projection from a Study of Large, Prepaid Group Practices," *JAMA*, Vol. 261, No. 13, 1989, pp. 1930-1934.

Mullan, F., M. L. Rivo, and R. M. Politzer, "Doctors, Dollars, and Determination: Making Physician Work-Force Policy," *Health Affairs*, Supplement 1993, 1993, pp. 138-151.

National Amulatory Medical Care Survey (NAMCS), *Patient Visits, 1991 Documentation and Magetic Tape*, National Center for Health Statistics, Hyattsville, Maryland, various years (1989, 1990, 1991).

National Health and Nutrition Examination Survey (NHANES). *Vital and Health Statistics: Plan and Operation of the Third National Health and Nutrition Examination Survey, 1988-1994.* Series 1: Programs and Collection Procedures, No. 32, DHHS (PHS) 94-1308, National Center for Health Statistics, Hyattsville, Maryland, 1994.

National Health Interview Survey (NHIS). *Vital and Health Statistics: Current Estimates from the National Health Interview Survey, 1992.* Series 10: Data from the National Health Survey, No. 189, DHHS (PHS) 94-1517, National Center for Health Statistics, Hyattsville, Maryland, 1994.

National Hospital Discharge Survey (NHDS), *Data Tape Documentation and Magnetic Tape*, National Center for Health Statistics, Hyattsville, Maryland, various years (1986, 1988, 1989, 1990).

Powell, W., "Medicare Cracks Down on Physician Retainers," *Argus*, July 1991, p. 12.

Prevent Blindness America, private correspondence, 1994.

Reinecke, R. D., "Ophthalmology Manpower Studies for the United States (Part I)," *Ophthalmology*, Vol. 85, 1978, pp. 1057-1137.

Reinecke, R. D., and T. Steinberg, "Manpower Studies for the United States: Part II Demand for Eye Care (A Public Opinion Poll Based Upon a Gallup Poll Survey)," *Ophthalmology*, Vol. 88, No. 4, 1981, pp. 34A-47A.

Reinhardt, U., "Manpower Substitution and Productivity in Medical Practice; Review of Research," *Health Services Research*, Fall 1973, pp. 201-227.

Reuben, D. B., J. Zwanziger, et al., "Projecting the Need for Physicians to Care for Older Persons: Effects of Changes in Demography, Utilization Patterns, and Physician Productivity," *JAGS*, Vol. 41, No. 10, 1993, pp. 1033-38.

Rivo, M. L., D. M. Jackson, and F. L. Clare, "Comparing Physician Workforce Reform Recommendations," *JAMA*, Vol. 270, No. 9, 1993, pp. 1083-84.

Rivo, M. L., and D. Satcher, "Improving Access to Health Care through Physician Workforce Reform," *JAMA*, Vol. 270, No. 9, 1993, pp. 1074-78.

Ruiz, R. S., "American Academy of Ophthalmology Manpower Studies: Part V," *Ophthalmology*, Vol. 91, No. 10, 1984, pp. 47A-57A.

Schroeder, S. A., "The Latest Forecast: Managed Care Collides with Physician Supply (Editorial)," *JAMA*, Vol. 272, No. 3, 1994, pp. 222-230.

Schwartz, W. B., F. A. Sloan, and D. N. Mendelson, "Why There Will Be Little or No Physician Surplus Between Now and the Year 2000," *NEJM*, Vol. 318, No. 14, 1988, pp. 892--897.

Singer, A. M., "Projections of Physician Supply and Demand: A Summary of HRSA and AMA Studies," *Academic Medicine*, Vol. 64, No. 5, 1989, pp. 235-240.

Southern California College of Optometry (SCCO), *The Future is in Sight, 1993-95 Catalog*, Fullerton, California, 1993.

Steinberg, E. P., E. B. Bass, K. Luthra, et al., "Normal Variation in Pre-Operative Ophthalmic Testing of Cataract Surgery Patients by Ophthalmologists," *Investigative Ophthalmology and Visual Science*, Vol. 34, No. 4, 1993, p. 1452.

U.S. Bureau of the Census, *Public Use Microdata Sample* (PUMS), 1990.

Walls, L. L., J. March, and M. Lapolla, "A Survey of Eye and Vision Care in Oklahoma," *Journal of the American Optometric Association*, Vol. 64, No. 11, 1993, pp. 799-808.

Weiner, J., "Forecasting the Effects of Health Reform on U. S. Physician Workforce Requirement: Evidence from HMO Staffing Patterns," *JAMA*, Vol. 272, No. 3, 1994, pp. 222-230.

Wennberg, J. E., D. C. Goodman, R. F. Nease, and R. B. Keller, "Finding Equilibrium in U. S. Physician Supply," *Health Affairs*, Vol. 12, No. 2, Summer 1993, pp. 89-103.

Worthen, D. M., M. N. Luxemberg, F. H. Gutman, et al., "Ophthalmology (Eye Physician and Surgeon) Manpower Studies for the United States: Part III A Survey of Ophthalmologists' Viewpoints and Practice Characteristics," *Ophthalmology*, Vol 88, No. 10, 1981, pp. 45A-51A.